Anti-Inflammatory Diet Cookbook for Beginners

Heal Your Body and Reduce Inflammation with Tasty Recipes and 30-Day Healthy Habits Meal Plan for Enhanced Immune System Health

By Vera Rice

Disclaimer

This cookbook and its content are provided for informational purposes only and are not intended to be medical advice or to replace the advice of a qualified healthcare professional. While the anti-inflammatory diet has been shown to benefit health in various ways, individual needs and responses to specific foods or dietary patterns can vary. Before beginning any new diet or making significant changes to your existing diet, please consult with a healthcare professional, especially if you have underlying health conditions or dietary restrictions.

The recipes and meal plans provided in this book are based on general principles of the anti-inflammatory diet and are intended to inspire healthier eating habits. They should not be considered as a one-size-fits-all solution for health issues related to inflammation or other medical conditions. The author and publisher have made every effort to ensure the accuracy of the information herein, but they cannot guarantee the outcomes of following the recommendations provided.

Neither the publisher nor the author shall be liable for any physical, psychological, emotional, financial, or commercial damages, including, but not limited to, special, incidental, consequential, or other damages. Readers should conduct their own due diligence and are solely responsible for their dietary choices and the preparation and consumption of the recipes contained in this book.

Table of Contents

Introduction

Embarking on a journey towards better health can often feel like navigating through a dense forest without a compass. With the plethora of dietary advice and health trends flooding our information channels, it's easy to feel lost and unsure where to begin. This is where the "Anti-Inflammatory Cookbook for Beginners" aims to make a difference. Designed with simplicity and accessibility in mind, this cookbook as your guide you through the complex landscape of nutritional health, steering you towards a path of wellness that is both achievable and grounded in scientific understanding.

Chronic inflammation is at the heart of many modern health issues, silently contributing to a range of diseases from cardiovascular disorders and diabetes to arthritis and beyond. The good news is that the power to combat this inflammation can be found at the end of your fork. The choices we make about what to put on our plates have a profound impact on our body's inflammatory responses. This cookbook is based on the principle that food should not only nourish and delight us but also serve as medicine to heal and protect our bodies.

Within these pages, you'll find an easy-to-follow introduction to the anti-inflammatory diet, a carefully curated selection of delicious recipes, and practical advice to make healthy eating a sustainable part of your lifestyle. Each recipe is designed with beginners in mind, ensuring that even those new to the kitchen can easily create nourishing meals. From hearty breakfasts and energizing snacks to satisfying mains and delightful desserts, these dishes leverage the power of anti-inflammatory ingredients to bring balance and health into your daily routine.

But this book is more than just a collection of recipes. It's an invitation to transform your health through the foods you enjoy every day. Alongside the recipes, you'll find insights into the science of inflammation, tips for stocking your anti-inflammatory pantry, and guidance on how to adapt recipes to suit your tastes and nutritional needs.

Whether you're looking to mitigate the risk of chronic disease, improve your energy levels and mental clarity, or embrace a more healthful way of eating, the "Anti-Inflammatory Cookbook for Beginners" is your first step on the journey towards a revitalized and inflammation-free life. Welcome to the beginning of your transformation.

Part 1: The Anti-Inflammatory Diet Basics

Understanding Inflammation

What is Inflammation?

Inflammation is a fundamental physiological process—a complex biological response of the body's immune system to harmful stimuli, such as pathogens (like bacteria and viruses), damaged cells (from injuries or conditions), or irritants. It is a protective mechanism, crucial for survival, that initiates the healing process by removing harmful stimuli and beginning the repair of affected tissues.

The Inflammatory Process

The process of inflammation can be broken down into several key stages:
- Recognition of Harmful Stimuli: The body's immune cells recognize the presence of harmful stimuli through various receptors. This recognition triggers an immune response aimed at neutralizing or eliminating the threat.
- Release of Inflammatory Mediators: Once harmful stimuli are detected, the body releases various substances, including histamines, cytokines, and prostaglandins. These mediators increase the permeability of blood vessels, allowing immune cells and nutrients to reach the affected site more easily.
- Recruitment of Immune Cells: Blood flow to the affected area increases, facilitating the arrival of immune cells like neutrophils and macrophages. These cells work to eliminate the harmful agents through phagocytosis (engulfing and digesting foreign particles) and to begin the healing process.
- Resolution of Inflammation: Ideally, once the harmful stimuli have been neutralized and the damaged tissue begins to heal, the inflammatory process resolves. Anti-inflammatory signals are released, helping to stop the inflammation and start the repair and regeneration of tissues.

Types of Inflammation

Inflammation can be classified into two main types based on its duration and characteristics:
- Acute Inflammation: This is a rapid response to an injury or infection, marked by local redness, heat, swelling, pain, and sometimes loss of function. Acute inflammation is typically a beneficial and necessary process that promotes healing. It usually resolves upon removing the initial cause or after the infected cells and tissues have been repaired.
- Chronic Inflammation: Unlike acute inflammation, chronic inflammation is a prolonged, often low-grade state that persists for months or even years. It can result from the inability to eliminate the cause of an acute inflammatory response, exposure to a low-level irritant over time, or an autoimmune reaction where the body's immune system mistakenly attacks healthy tissue. Chronic inflammation is associated with various diseases, such as heart disease, diabetes, cancer, arthritis, and neurodegenerative conditions like Alzheimer's disease.

Causes of Inflammation

The causes of inflammation are varied and can be broadly categorized into several key areas:

1. Infections

Infections by microorganisms, including bacteria, viruses, fungi, and parasites, are common causes of inflammation. The body's immune system detects these foreign invaders and responds by activating inflammatory pathways to isolate and eliminate the infection, often resulting in symptoms such as fever, swelling, and redness.

2. Physical Injuries

Physical trauma to the body, such as cuts, burns, fractures, sprains, or blunt force, can lead to acute inflammation. This response is part of the body's natural healing process, involving the release of inflammatory mediators to start the repair of damaged tissue.

3. Foreign Bodies

The presence of foreign bodies, such as splinters, dust, or other non-biological irritants, can trigger an inflammatory response. The body recognizes these objects as potential threats and initiates inflammation to neutralize and remove them.

4. Toxins

Exposure to certain chemicals and environmental pollutants can cause inflammation. This includes exposure to toxic substances from industrial chemicals, air and water pollutants, and certain household cleaners. Even lifestyle factors such as smoking, excessive alcohol consumption, and a diet high in processed foods can introduce toxins into the body, leading to inflammation.

5. Autoimmune Disorders

In autoimmune disorders, the immune system mistakenly identifies healthy cells and tissues as harmful, leading to an inflammatory response against the body's own cells. This can result in diseases such as rheumatoid arthritis, lupus, and type 1 diabetes, where chronic inflammation plays a key role.

6. Chronic Conditions and Lifestyle Factors

Certain chronic conditions, such as obesity, metabolic syndrome, and type 2 diabetes, are closely linked to chronic inflammation. These conditions can alter the body's metabolic processes and immune responses, leading to persistent inflammation. Additionally, lifestyle factors like sedentary behavior, chronic stress, and poor sleep habits can contribute to the development and exacerbation of chronic inflammation.

7. Dietary Factors

The diet plays a significant role in influencing inflammation. Diets high in saturated fats, trans fats, sugars, and refined carbohydrates can promote inflammation, while diets rich in fruits, vegetables, whole grains, lean proteins, and healthy fats (such as fish and olive oil) can help reduce inflammation.

Understanding the difference between acute and chronic inflammation is crucial for recognizing how dietary choices and lifestyle changes can influence our health. By adopting an anti-inflammatory diet, which will be explored in the subsequent chapters of this cookbook, individuals can take proactive steps toward reducing chronic inflammation and enhancing their overall well-being.

Through the recipes and guidance provided in this cookbook, readers will learn how to incorporate anti-inflammatory foods into their daily meals, potentially reducing their risk of chronic diseases and improving their quality of life.

The Role of Diet in Managing Inflammation

The connection between diet and inflammation is profound and well-documented. While inflammation is a natural immune response necessary for healing, chronic inflammation can lead to numerous health issues, including heart disease, diabetes, arthritis, and various autoimmune diseases. The foods we consume play a significant role in either fueling or fighting inflammation.

Foods That Exacerbate Inflammation

Foods that exacerbate inflammation do so through various biological mechanisms, including promoting oxidative stress, altering gut microbiota, and triggering immune system responses. Consuming these foods in high quantities or regularly can contribute to chronic inflammation associated with an increased risk of various diseases. Here is a more detailed look at these pro-inflammatory foods:

1. Refined Carbohydrates

Refined carbohydrates are processed foods from which the fiber and nutrients have been removed. Examples include white bread, rice, pastries, and other baked goods made from refined flour. These foods have a high glycemic index, which means they cause a rapid spike in blood sugar levels. High blood sugar levels can lead to an overproduction of inflammatory cytokines and a reduction in blood vessel function, contributing to inflammatory responses throughout the body.

2. Sugar

Sugar is a major dietary contributor to inflammation, particularly in its refined form as sucrose (table sugar) and high-fructose corn syrup. Found in a wide range of processed foods, from sodas and candies to baked goods and even some savory items, excessive sugar intake can lead to obesity, insulin resistance, and diabetes, all of which are associated with increased levels of inflammation. Sugar stimulates the production of fatty acids in the liver, which can trigger inflammatory processes.

3. Saturated and Trans-Fats

Saturated fats, found in animal products like red meat, butter, and cheese, as well as some tropical oils, can activate inflammatory pathways, specifically through the activation of toll-like receptors (TLRs) on immune cells. Trans fats, which are created through hydrogenation and found in margarine, fried foods, and many processed foods, can increase LDL cholesterol (the "bad" cholesterol) and decrease HDL cholesterol (the "good" cholesterol), leading to inflammation of the arteries and increasing the risk of heart disease.

4. Omega-6 Fatty Acids

While omega-6 fatty acids are essential for health, an imbalance between omega-6 and omega-3 fatty acids in the diet can promote inflammation. Modern diets often have a high ratio of omega-6s to omega-3s, contributing to inflammatory processes. Omega-6 fatty acids are found in certain vegetable oils (such as corn, sunflower, and soybean oils) and processed foods made with these oils.

5. Alcohol

Moderate alcohol consumption might have some health benefits, but excessive intake is harmful and can lead to inflammation. Alcohol can damage liver cells, leading to inflammation as the body attempts to repair the damage. Over time, chronic alcohol consumption can lead to persistent inflammation, increasing the risk of liver diseases, including fatty liver disease and cirrhosis

6. Processed Meat

Processed meats, such as sausages, bacon, ham, and deli meats, contain high levels of saturated fats, advanced glycation end products (AGEs), and certain additives that can promote inflammation. The consumption of processed meats has been linked to an increased risk of chronic diseases, including heart disease and cancer, partly due to their inflammatory effects.

Understanding the inflammatory potential of these foods can help guide dietary choices toward more anti-inflammatory options. While it's not necessary to eliminate these foods entirely, reducing their intake and balancing them with nutrient-dense, anti-inflammatory foods can significantly impact managing inflammation and overall health.

Foods That Reduce Inflammation

Foods that reduce inflammation do so by providing antioxidants, polyphenols, omega-3 fatty acids, fiber, and various phytonutrients that help neutralize free radicals, decrease the production of pro-inflammatory cytokines, and promote a healthy immune response. Incorporating these foods into one's diet can help manage, reduce, or even prevent chronic inflammation. Here's a closer look at these anti-inflammatory foods:

1. Omega-3 Fatty Acids

Omega-3 fatty acids are known for their potent anti-inflammatory properties. They are found in high concentrations in fatty fish like salmon, mackerel, sardines, and anchovies. Plant sources include flaxseeds, chia seeds, hemp seeds, and walnuts. Omega-3s help reduce the production of molecules and substances linked to inflammation, such as eicosanoids and cytokines.

2. Fruits and Vegetables

Fruits and vegetables are rich sources of antioxidants, vitamins, minerals, and fiber, which can help combat inflammation. Some of the most potent anti-inflammatory fruits and vegetables include:

- Berries: Strawberries, blueberries, raspberries, and blackberries are packed with vitamins, minerals, and antioxidants called anthocyanins that have anti-inflammatory effects.
- Leafy Greens: Spinach, kale, and collard greens are high in vitamin E and other powerful antioxidants that help protect the body from pro-inflammatory molecules called cytokines.

- Cruciferous Vegetables: Broccoli, cauliflower, brussels sprouts, and cabbage contain sulforaphane, an antioxidant that fights inflammation by reducing levels of cytokines and NF-kB, a molecule that drives inflammation.

3. Whole Grains

Whole grains like brown rice, quinoa, whole wheat, oats, and barley are rich in fiber, which has been shown to reduce levels of C-reactive protein (CRP), a blood inflammation marker. They also provide essential minerals and B vitamins that support a healthy inflammatory response.

4. Nuts and Seeds

Nuts and seeds are excellent sources of healthy fats, protein, fiber, antioxidants, and anti-inflammatory compounds. Almonds and walnuts, in particular, are high in omega-3 fatty acids, vitamin E, and magnesium. Similarly, seeds like flaxseeds, chia seeds, and hemp seeds offer significant amounts of omega-3s and antioxidants.

5. Spices and Herbs

Many spices and herbs are loaded with antioxidants, offering significant anti-inflammatory benefits:
- Turmeric: Contains curcumin, a compound with potent anti-inflammatory and antioxidant properties. Curcumin is especially effective in reducing inflammation related to arthritis, diabetes, and other diseases.
- Ginger: Has gingerol, which inhibits the synthesis of pro-inflammatory cytokines and helps reduce pain and soreness.
- Garlic: Contains allicin and diallyl disulfide, compounds that have been shown to reduce inflammation, fight infection, and boost the immune system.

6. Extra Virgin Olive Oil

Extra virgin olive oil is a foundational element of diets focused on reducing inflammation, celebrated for its cardiovascular benefits and potent anti-inflammatory properties. It contains oleocanthal, a unique compound with effects comparable to those of ibuprofen, an anti-inflammatory medication. Additionally, olive oil is an excellent source of monounsaturated fats, which play a crucial role in diminishing inflammation throughout the body.

7. Dark Chocolate and Cocoa

Dark chocolate and cocoa are packed with antioxidants known as flavonoids, which may reduce inflammation. Choosing dark chocolate with a high cocoa content (at least 70%) is essential to maximize the benefits and limit added sugar.

Incorporating these anti-inflammatory foods into your diet can help reduce the risk of chronic inflammation and related diseases. A diet centered around whole, nutrient-dense foods supports overall health and provides a natural defense against inflammation.

The Anti-Inflammatory Diet: Principles and Practices

An anti-inflammatory diet focuses on whole, nutrient-dense foods while minimizing processed products and sugars. The Mediterranean diet is often cited as an exemplary model of an anti-inflammatory eating pattern due to its emphasis on fruits, vegetables, whole grains, fatty fish, and healthy oils.

Managing inflammation through diet involves mindful choices and focusing on whole, natural foods. By understanding foods' inflammatory or anti-inflammatory properties, individuals can better manage their health, potentially reducing their risk of chronic diseases associated with chronic inflammation. This cookbook aims to provide recipes that harness the power of anti-inflammatory ingredients, making it easier for beginners to adopt a healthful eating pattern that supports long-term well-being.

In the following chapters, we will explore delicious, simple recipes to incorporate these anti-inflammatory foods into your daily meals, helping you embrace a lifestyle that naturally combats inflammation.

Deciphering Food Labels: Identifying Inflammatory Ingredients

Understanding how to read food labels is critical to adopting an anti-inflammatory diet. The marketplace is flooded with products claiming to be healthy, but a closer examination of their labels often reveals the presence of ingredients that could contribute to inflammation. This subchapter aims to teach you to discern truly healthful foods from those that might undermine your anti-inflammatory eating efforts.

The Basics of Food Labels

Before diving into specific ingredients, it's essential to understand the structure of food labels. Most packaged foods feature a Nutrition Facts panel, which lists critical nutritional information, including calories, fats, carbohydrates, and proteins per serving. Below this panel, you'll find an ingredients list, where items are presented in descending order by weight. This means that the first few ingredients make up the bulk of the product, a crucial detail when assessing a food's potential inflammatory impact.

Common Inflammatory Ingredients

Refined Sugars:

- Names to Look For: High-fructose corn syrup, dextrose, sucrose, maltose, and other terms ending in "-ose."
- Why to Avoid: These sugars can spike blood sugar levels, leading to inflammation.

Trans and Saturated Fats:

- Names to Look For: Partially hydrogenated oils, hydrogenated oils, palm oil, and lard.
- Why to Avoid: These fats can increase bad cholesterol levels and trigger inflammatory responses.

Artificial Additives:

- Names to Look For: Monosodium glutamate (MSG), artificial flavors, colors, and sweeteners like aspartame.
- Why to Avoid: Such additives can disrupt the gut microbiome and contribute to inflammation.

Omega-6 Fatty Acids in Excess:

- Names to Look For: Vegetable oils like corn, soybean, and sunflower.
- Why to Avoid: While necessary in small amounts, an imbalance between omega-6 and omega-3 fatty acids in the diet can promote inflammation.

Tips for Avoiding Inflammatory Ingredients

- Prioritize Whole Foods: The less processed a food is, the less likely it is to contain inflammatory ingredients.
- Learn Synonyms: Sugar, fats, and additives often appear under numerous names. Please familiarize yourself with these to better spot them.
- Check the Serving Size: Sometimes, unhealthy ingredients appear minor due to the small serving sizes listed. Assess portions realistically.
- Opt for Short Ingredients Lists: Generally, foods with fewer ingredients are less processed and healthier.

Mastering reading food labels is a powerful tool in maintaining an anti-inflammatory diet. By learning to identify and avoid foods with inflammatory ingredients, you can make choices that support your health and well-being. Remember, the goal is not perfection but progress as you gradually shift towards a diet rich in whole, nutrient-dense foods that nurture rather than inflame your body.

Goals of the Cookbook:

Enhancing Overall Health through Dietary Transformation

The foremost ambition of this cookbook is to catalyze profound improvements in your health by focusing on reducing inflammation—a condition at the heart of many chronic diseases and health issues. Chronic inflammation has been linked to a host of ailments, from cardiovascular diseases and diabetes to autoimmune conditions and beyond. This cookbook aims to guide you toward a dietary pattern that minimizes the factors contributing to inflammation, potentially mitigating the risk of these conditions. Through carefully curated recipes and nutritional insights, we strive to promote a balanced, nutrient-rich diet that supports the body's immune system, enhances metabolic health, and fosters overall well-being.

Demystifying Healthy Cooking with Accessible Recipes

Understanding the challenges of adopting new dietary habits, especially for those with minimal cooking experience or limited time, this cookbook prioritizes simplicity and accessibility in its recipes. Each recipe is designed to demystify the cooking process, presenting clear, concise instructions paired with tips for ingredient substitutions and kitchen hacks to streamline cooking. The goal is to make healthy eating achievable and enjoyable for everyone, regardless of their culinary skill level. By breaking down barriers to healthy cooking, we aim to empower readers to confidently prepare meals that are not only nourishing but also delicious and satisfying.

Introducing a Comprehensive Approach to Anti-Inflammatory Eating

Central to this cookbook is introducing an anti-inflammatory diet as a holistic approach to health. Unlike restrictive diets that focus narrowly on weight loss or calorie counting, the anti-inflammatory diet emphasizes food's quality and nutritional value. This cookbook will showcase various ingredients known for their anti-inflammatory properties—such as omega-3-rich fish, colorful fruits and vegetables packed with antioxidants, whole grains full of fiber, and healthy fats from nuts, seeds, and olive oil. The recipes and guidance provided will illustrate how to integrate these foods into daily meals in a way that is both healthful and flavorful, aiming to inspire a long-term dietary shift rather than a temporary change.

The journey through this cookbook is intended to be enlightening, empowering, and transformative, providing a collection of recipes and a blueprint for a healthier way of life. By aligning with the above goals, readers will embark toward improved health, armed with the culinary skills and nutritional knowledge necessary to combat inflammation. Ultimately, this cookbook aims to inspire a dietary and lifestyle shift that fosters vitality, well-being, and a deeper connection to the healing power of food.

Part 2: Getting Started

Kitchen Essentials: Guide to Stocking Your Kitchen for Anti-Inflammatory Meals

Embarking on an anti-inflammatory diet journey is as much about what you eat as it is about how you prepare your meals. A well-stocked kitchen with the right tools and pantry staples is your foundation for creating nourishing, anti-inflammatory meals with ease. This guide outlines the essentials every beginner should have on hand, ensuring you're always ready to whip up something wholesome and delicious.

Essential Kitchen Tools

Creating anti-inflammatory meals doesn't require fancy gadgets, but a few essential tools can make the process more efficient and enjoyable:
- Chef's Knife: A sharp, versatile knife for chopping vegetables, fruits, and herbs.
- Cutting Board: Opt for a large, durable board for ample prep space.
- Blender or Food Processor: Ideal for smoothies, soups, and sauces packed with anti-inflammatory ingredients.
- Non-Stick Skillet and Pots: Look for quality cookware for sautéing vegetables and simmering grains.
- Measuring Cups and Spoons: Essential for following recipes accurately.
- Mixing Bowls: A set of various sizes for mixing and tossing ingredients.
- Storage Containers: Glass or BPA-free plastic containers for storing leftovers and prepped ingredients.

Pantry Staples

A pantry well-stocked with anti-inflammatory staples ensures you always have the base for a healthy meal at your fingertips:
- Whole Grains: Quinoa, brown rice, and oats provide fiber and nutrients.
- Legumes: Beans, lentils, and chickpeas are excellent plant-based protein sources.
- Healthy Fats: Extra virgin olive oil, coconut oil, and avocado oil for cooking and dressings.
- Nuts and Seeds: Almonds, walnuts, chia seeds, and flaxseeds offer healthy fats and texture.
- Herbs and Spices: Turmeric, ginger, garlic, and cinnamon for flavor and anti-inflammatory benefits.
- Canned Goods: Low-sodium canned tomatoes and light coconut milk for convenience without sacrificing health.
- Vinegar and Sauces: Apple cider vinegar and low-sodium soy sauce or tamari for depth of flavor.
- Sweeteners: Opt for natural sweeteners like honey or pure maple syrup in moderation.

Refrigerator and Freezer Staples

Keep your refrigerator and freezer stocked with fresh and frozen produce and proteins:

- Fresh Vegetables and Fruits: A variety of colors to maximize nutrient intake.
- Lean Proteins: Chicken, turkey, and fish like salmon and mackerel.
- Frozen Produce: Berries, spinach, and broccoli for smoothies and quick meals.
- Dairy Alternatives: Almond, coconut, or oat milk for those avoiding dairy.

Equipping your kitchen with these essentials sets the stage for successful anti-inflammatory cooking. With the right tools and various pantry staples, you can easily incorporate anti-inflammatory meals into your daily routine. Remember, the journey to better health through food is a marathon, not a sprint. Start with the basics, and gradually build your kitchen to reflect the diversity and richness of the anti-inflammatory diet.

Meal Planning and Prep: Strategies for a Nutrient-Rich Week

Embracing an anti-inflammatory diet is more than just a daily decision—it's about creating a sustainable lifestyle. A crucial component of this lifestyle is meal planning and prep. Effective meal planning ensures that you're consuming a wide array of nutrients and enjoying a variety of flavors, all while minimizing stress and saving time. This subchapter offers practical strategies to help you organize your meals throughout the week, making healthy eating accessible and delightful.

Step 1: Understanding Your Nutritional Goals

Begin by familiarizing yourself with the key components of an anti-inflammatory diet—whole grains, lean proteins, healthy fats, and a rainbow of fruits and vegetables. Your goal is to incorporate these elements into your weekly meals in a balanced and enjoyable way.

Step 2: Meal Planning Basics

Create a Weekly Meal Plan:

- Sketch out a week: Outline your weekly meals, including breakfast, lunch, dinner, and snacks. Consider your schedule and plan simpler meals for busier days.

Diversify your menu:

- Ensure variety by including proteins, grains, and vegetables throughout the week. This keeps meals interesting and covers a broad spectrum of nutrients.

Compile Your Shopping List:

- Organize by category: Make your shopping list based on the layout of your grocery store (produce, proteins, dairy, etc.) to streamline your shopping trip.
- Stick to the list: This helps you avoid impulse buys that might not align with your anti-inflammatory goals.

Step 3: Meal Prep Strategies

Batch Cooking:

- Cook once, eat multiple times: Prepare large batches of staples like grains, proteins, and roasted vegetables at the beginning of the week. Use these as the base for various meals to save time.

Utilize Leftovers Creatively:

- Reinvent meals: Transform leftovers into new dishes to keep things interesting. For example, last night's roasted chicken can become today's chicken salad.

Prepping Ingredients:

- Chop and store: Wash, chop, and store vegetables and fruits in clear containers for easy weekly access. This makes throwing together a meal or snack much quicker.

Step 4: Implementing Your Plan

Set Aside Time:

- Dedicate prep time: Block off a few hours one day a week for meal prep. This upfront investment of time saves you hours over the week and keeps you on track with healthy eating.

Stay Flexible:

- Adapt as needed: Life is unpredictable. Have quick, healthy backup options for those days when things don't go as planned, such as frozen vegetables or pre-cooked proteins.

Meal planning and prep are not about strict adherence to a set schedule but about making the anti-inflammatory lifestyle as seamless and enjoyable as possible. Investing a little time in planning and prep ensures a week filled with nutritious, anti-inflammatory meals that support your health and fit your busy lifestyle. Remember, the key is balance and flexibility, allowing you to enjoy the wide array of flavors and nutrients that an anti-inflammatory diet offers.

Tips for Beginners: Mastering the Basics of Anti-Inflammatory Cooking

Embarking on a journey toward better health through anti-inflammatory cooking can be exciting and daunting. This subchapter is designed to ease you into the process, offering practical advice on simple cooking techniques, savvy grocery shopping, and making meal prep a seamless part of your routine. With these tips, you'll find that preparing nourishing, delicious meals can be straightforward and deeply satisfying.

Simple Cooking Techniques

Embrace the Basics:

- Stir-frying: Quickly cook vegetables and lean proteins in a small amount of healthy fat like olive or avocado oil. This method retains nutrients and concentrates flavors.
- Roasting: Roasting vegetables, fruits, and proteins at a high temperature enhances natural sweetness and complexity with minimal effort.
- Steaming: Preserve the nutritional content of vegetables by steaming them until just tender. It's a quick, easy method that requires minimal equipment.

Flavor with Anti-Inflammatory Spices:

- Incorporate spices such as turmeric, ginger, and garlic into your dishes. These add depth of flavor and significant anti-inflammatory benefits without extra calories or sodium.

Grocery Shopping Tips

Plan Ahead:

- Create a shopping list based on your meal plan for the week. Stick to your list to avoid impulse buys that aren't in line with your anti-inflammatory goals.

Shop the Perimeter:

- Most stores lay out healthier, whole-food options along the perimeter. Start there to fill your cart with fresh produce, proteins, and dairy alternatives before heading to the inner aisles for pantry staples.

Read Labels Carefully:

- When purchasing packaged foods, read the ingredients list. Look for short lists with recognizable ingredients and avoid products with added sugars, trans fats, and artificial additives.

Making Meal Prep Efficient and Enjoyable

Set a Prep Day:

- Choose a day each week to do most of your meal prep. Cooking in batches can save time and ensure you have healthy options readily available.

Invest in Quality Containers:

- Suitable storage containers are worth their weight in gold for keeping prepped ingredients and leftovers fresh. Opt for glass or BPA-free plastic that can go from fridge to microwave.

Involve Family or Friends:

- Meal prep doesn't have to be a solitary task. Involve your household or make it a social occasion with friends. Cooking together can be fun to share the workload and enjoy the process.

Anti-inflammatory cooking is not just about following recipes; it's about incorporating new habits into your lifestyle. By mastering a few simple cooking techniques, becoming a savvy shopper, and making meal prep a regular, enjoyable part of your week, you'll be well on your way to enjoying the myriad benefits of an anti-inflammatory diet. Remember, the goal is progress, not perfection. Each step you take is a step towards better health.

Part 3: Recipes

Breakfast

Golden Turmeric Porridge

Yield: 4 servings | **Prep time:** 5 minutes | **Cook time:** 15 minutes

Ingredients:

- 1 cup rolled oats (can be replaced with gluten-free oatmeal)
- 2 cups unsweetened almond milk
- 1 cup water
- 1 tablespoon ground turmeric
- 1 teaspoon ground cinnamon
- 1/4 teaspoon ground ginger
- 1/4 teaspoon black pepper (to enhance turmeric absorption)
- 2 tablespoons maple syrup (or to taste)
- 1/2 cup fresh blueberries
- 1/4 cup chopped walnuts
- Optional toppings: sliced bananas, a dollop of almond butter

Nutritional Information: Estimated 210 calories, 6g protein, 35g carbohydrates, 7g fat, 6g fiber, 0mg cholesterol, 30mg sodium, 200mg potassium.

Directions:

1. Combine the rolled oats, almond milk, water, turmeric, cinnamon, ginger, and black pepper in a medium saucepan. Bring to a simmer over medium heat, stirring frequently.
2. Reduce heat to low and cook for 10-15 minutes until the porridge has thickened to your liking, stirring occasionally to prevent sticking.
3. Remove from heat and stir in the maple syrup. Adjust sweetness to taste.
4. Serve the porridge hot, garnished with fresh blueberries, chopped walnuts, and any additional toppings you choose.

Chia and Hemp Seed Superfood Pudding

Yield: 4 servings | **Prep time:** 10 minutes | **Cook time:** 0 minutes (plus at least 4 hours of refrigeration)

Ingredients:

- 1/4 cup chia seeds
- 1/4 cup hemp seeds
- 2 cups unsweetened almond milk
- 1 tablespoon pure maple syrup (adjust to taste)
- 1 teaspoon vanilla extract
- Fresh berries for topping (such as strawberries, blueberries, or raspberries)
- Optional: a pinch of cinnamon or ground cardamom for flavor

Nutritional Information: Estimated 220 calories, 10g protein, 12g carbohydrates, 15g fat, 10g fiber, 0mg cholesterol, 30mg sodium, 200mg potassium.

Directions:

1. Whisk together the chia seeds, hemp seeds, almond milk, maple syrup, and vanilla extract in a medium mixing bowl. If desired, add a pinch of cinnamon or cardamom for extra flavor.
2. Divide the mixture evenly among four serving bowls or mason jars. Cover and refrigerate for at least 4 hours, or overnight, until the pudding thickens and the chia seeds fully absorb the liquid.
3. Before serving, stir the pudding to ensure it has a uniform consistency. Top with fresh berries of your choice.

Avocado and Egg Breakfast Bowl

Yield: 2 servings | **Prep time:** 5 minutes | **Cook time:** 10 minutes

Ingredients:

- 2 large eggs
- 1 ripe avocado, halved and sliced
- 2 cups baby spinach
- 1/2 cup cooked quinoa
- 1 tablespoon olive oil
- Salt and pepper to taste
- Optional garnish: cherry tomatoes, cut, and a sprinkle of chia seeds

Nutritional Information: Estimated 350 calories, 14g protein, 22g carbohydrates, 24g fat, 10g fiber, 186mg cholesterol, 200mg sodium, 800mg potassium.

Directions:

1. Heat the olive oil in a skillet over medium heat. Add the baby spinach and sauté until just wilted, about 2-3 minutes—season with salt and pepper to taste. Divide the spinach between two bowls.
2. In the same skillet, cook the eggs to your liking (poached, fried, or scrambled).
3. Divide the cooked quinoa and sliced avocado between the bowls, arranging them alongside the wilted spinach.
4. Top each bowl with a cooked egg. Garnish with cherry tomatoes and a sprinkle of chia seeds if desired.

Ginger Infused Mixed Berry Smoothie

Yield: 2 servings | **Prep time:** 5 minutes | **Cook time:** 0 minutes

Ingredients:

- 1 cup frozen mixed berries (strawberries, blueberries, raspberries, and blackberries)
- 1 medium banana, sliced
- 1/2 inch fresh ginger, peeled and minced
- 1 cup spinach leaves
- 1 tablespoon chia seeds
- 1 cup unsweetened almond milk
- Optional: 1 tablespoon honey or maple syrup for added sweetness

Nutritional Information: Estimated 180 calories, 4g protein, 35g carbohydrates, 3g fat, 8g fiber, 0mg cholesterol, 80mg sodium, 400mg potassium.

Directions:

1. Place the frozen mixed berries, banana slices, minced ginger, spinach leaves, chia seeds, and almond milk into a blender. Add honey or maple syrup if you prefer a sweeter taste.
2. Blend on high until smooth and creamy. Add more almond milk to reach your desired consistency if the smoothie is too thick.
3. Taste and adjust sweetness if necessary, blending again if you add more sweetener.
4. Pour the smoothie into glasses and serve immediately for the best flavor and nutrient retention.

Cinnamon Spiced Baked Apples with Walnuts

Yield: 4 servings | **Prep time:** 10 minutes | **Cook time:** 30 minutes

Ingredients:

- 4 large apples, such as Honeycrisp or Granny Smith, cored
- 1/4 cup chopped walnuts
- 2 tablespoons pure maple syrup
- 1/2 teaspoon ground cinnamon
- 1/4 teaspoon ground nutmeg
- 1/4 cup raisins (optional)
- 1 cup unsweetened apple juice or water

Nutritional Information: Estimated 200 calories, 2g protein, 40g carbohydrates, 5g fat, 6g fiber, 0mg cholesterol, 5mg sodium, 300mg potassium.

Directions:

1. Preheat your oven to 350°F (175°C). Arrange the cored apples in a baking dish that fits them snugly.
2. Mix the chopped walnuts, maple syrup, ground cinnamon, ground nutmeg, and raisins (if using) in a small bowl. Spoon this mixture into the center of each apple.
3. Pour the apple juice or water into the bottom of the baking dish. This will help to steam the apples as they bake, keeping them moist.
4. Cover the dish with aluminum foil and bake in the preheated oven for about 25 to 30 minutes or until the apples are tender when pierced with a fork.
5. Serve the baked apples warm, spooning some cooking liquid from the dish over the top.

Quinoa Breakfast Muffins

Yield: 6 servings | **Prep time:** 15 minutes | **Cook time:** 20 minutes

Ingredients:

- 1 cup cooked quinoa
- 1/2 cup almond flour
- 1/4 cup ground flaxseed
- 1 teaspoon baking powder
- 1/2 teaspoon cinnamon
- 1/4 teaspoon salt
- 2 large eggs
- 1/4 cup unsweetened almond milk
- 1/4 cup pure maple syrup
- 1 teaspoon vanilla extract
- 1/2 cup fresh blueberries
- 1/4 cup chopped walnuts

Nutritional Information: Estimated 220 calories, 8g protein, 28g carbohydrates, 10g fat, 5g fiber, 62mg cholesterol, 180mg sodium, 250mg potassium.

Directions:

1. Preheat your oven to 350°F (175 °C), line a muffin tin with paper liners, or grease it with coconut oil.
2. Mix the cooked quinoa, almond flour, ground flaxseed, baking powder, cinnamon, and salt in a large bowl.
3. Whisk together the eggs, almond milk, maple syrup, and vanilla extract in another bowl. Pour the wet ingredients into the dry ingredients, stirring until just combined. Fold in the blueberries and walnuts.
4. Divide the batter evenly among the prepared muffin cups, filling each about three-quarters full.
5. Bake for 20 minutes or until a toothpick inserted into the center of a muffin comes out clean. Let the muffins cool in the pan for 5 minutes before transferring them to a wire rack to cool completely.

Sweet Potato and Kale Hash with Poached Eggs

Yield: 4 servings | **Prep time:** 15 minutes | **Cook time:** 25 minutes

Ingredients:

- 2 medium sweet potatoes, peeled and diced
- 2 cups kale, washed and chopped
- 1 medium onion, diced
- 2 tablespoons olive oil
- 1 teaspoon smoked paprika
- Salt and pepper to taste
- 4 large eggs
- 2 tablespoons white vinegar (for poaching eggs)
- Optional garnish: fresh parsley, chopped

Nutritional Information: Estimated 300 calories, 10g protein, 35g carbohydrates, 14g fat, 6g fiber, 186mg cholesterol, 200mg sodium, 600mg potassium.

Directions:

1. Heat the olive oil in a large skillet over medium heat and sauté the diced onion until translucent, about 5 minutes. Add the diced sweet potatoes, smoked paprika, salt, and pepper, cooking until the sweet potatoes are tender, approximately 15 minutes.
2. Stir in the chopped kale until it wilts and becomes tender, about 3-5 minutes. Adjust seasoning as needed.
3. Meanwhile, bring a pot of water to a gentle simmer and add the white vinegar. Crack each egg into a small bowl and gently slide it into the simmering water. Poach the eggs for about 3-4 minutes, or until the whites are set but the yolks remain runny. Remove with a slotted spoon and drain on a paper towel.
4. Divide the sweet potato and kale hash among plates. Top each serving with a poached egg. Garnish with fresh parsley if desired.

Flaxseed and Banana Pancakes

Yield: 4 servings | **Prep time:** 10 minutes | **Cook time:** 15 minutes

Ingredients:

- 2 ripe bananas, mashed
- 2 eggs
- 1/2 cup almond milk
- 1 cup oat flour (can be replaced with gluten-free flour)
- 1/4 cup ground flaxseed
- 1 teaspoon baking powder
- 1/2 teaspoon cinnamon
- 1 teaspoon vanilla extract
- Coconut oil for cooking
- Optional toppings: fresh berries, almond butter, or a drizzle of maple syrup

Nutritional Information: Estimated 250 calories, 8g protein, 38g carbohydrates, 8g fat, 6g fiber, 93mg cholesterol, 150mg sodium, 350mg potassium.

Directions:

1. Combine the mashed bananas, eggs, almond milk, and vanilla extract in a large mixing bowl. Mix well until the mixture is smooth.
2. Whisk together the oat flour, ground flaxseed, baking powder, and cinnamon in another bowl. Gradually add the dry ingredients to the wet ingredients, stirring until combined.
3. Heat a skillet over medium heat and lightly grease with coconut oil. Pour 1/4 cup of batter for each pancake onto the skillet. Cook for 2-3 minutes on one side or until bubbles form on the surface, then flip and cook for 1-2 minutes on the other side.
4. Serve the pancakes warm with your choice of toppings.

Spinach, Feta, and Red Pepper Omelette

Yield: 2 servings | **Prep time:** 5 minutes | **Cook time:** 10 minutes

Ingredients:

- 4 large eggs
- 1/4 cup almond milk
- 1/2 cup fresh spinach, chopped
- 1/4 cup red bell pepper, diced
- 1/4 cup feta cheese, crumbled
- 1 tablespoon olive oil
- Salt and pepper to taste
- Optional garnish: fresh herbs (such as parsley or chives)

Nutritional Information: Estimated 300 calories, 20g protein, 6g carbohydrates, 22g fat, 1g fiber, 372mg cholesterol, 500mg sodium, 200mg potassium.

Directions:

1. Whisk together eggs, almond milk, salt, and pepper in a mixing bowl until well combined.
2. Heat olive oil in a non-stick skillet over medium heat. Add the diced red bell pepper and sauté for 2-3 minutes until slightly softened. Add the spinach and cook until just wilted, about 1-2 minutes.
3. Pour the egg mixture over the sautéed vegetables in the skillet, tilting the pan to ensure an even spread. Cook for 3-4 minutes or until the eggs set around the edges.
4. Sprinkle the crumbled feta cheese over half of the omelet. Use a spatula to fold the omelet in half, covering the cheese. Cook for another 1-2 minutes or until the cheese melts and the omelet is cooked to your liking.
5. Carefully slide the omelet onto a plate, garnish with fresh herbs if desired, and serve immediately.

Coconut Yogurt with Pomegranate and Almonds

Yield: 4 servings | **Prep time:** 5 minutes | **Cook time:** 0 minutes

Ingredients:

- 2 cups unsweetened coconut yogurt
- 1 cup pomegranate seeds
- 1/2 cup sliced almonds, toasted
- 2 tablespoons honey or maple syrup (optional)
- 1/2 teaspoon ground cinnamon

Nutritional Information: Estimated 250 calories, 6g protein, 18g carbohydrates, 18g fat, 5g fiber, 0mg cholesterol, 30mg sodium, 300mg potassium.

Directions:

1. In serving bowls, evenly distribute the coconut yogurt.
2. Top each bowl of yogurt with an equal amount of pomegranate seeds and toasted sliced almonds.
3. Drizzle with honey or maple syrup if a sweeter taste is desired.
4. Sprinkle ground cinnamon over each serving for added flavor.

Carrot and Ginger Warm Breakfast Salad

Yield: 4 servings | **Prep time:** 10 minutes | **Cook time:** 15 minutes

Ingredients:

- 4 large carrots, peeled and thinly sliced
- 2 tablespoons fresh ginger, minced
- 4 cups baby spinach leaves
- 1/4 cup raw walnuts, chopped
- 2 tablespoons olive oil
- 2 tablespoons apple cider vinegar
- 1 teaspoon honey (optional)
- Salt and pepper to taste
- 4 large eggs

Nutritional Information: Estimated 250 calories, 12g protein, 18g carbohydrates, 16g fat, 5g fiber, 185mg cholesterol, 220mg sodium, 600mg potassium.

Directions:

1. Heat 1 tablespoon of olive oil over medium heat in a large skillet. Add the minced ginger and sauté for about 1 minute until fragrant. Add the sliced carrots, salt, and pepper, and cook for about 5-7 minutes until they are tender but still have a slight crunch.
2. Add the spinach to the skillet, stirring until just wilted. Remove from heat and transfer the vegetable mixture to a serving bowl. Drizzle with apple cider vinegar and the remaining olive oil. Toss gently to combine. Sprinkle with chopped walnuts.
3. In the same skillet, reduce heat to medium-low. Crack the eggs into the skillet, careful not to break the yolks. Cook until the whites are set but the yolks are still runny, or to your preference. Season with salt and pepper.
4. Divide the warm salad among plates and top each with a fried egg. Drizzle with honey if desired for a touch of sweetness.

Broccoli and Quinoa Breakfast Casserole

Yield: 4 servings | **Prep time:** 15 minutes | **Cook time:** 30 minutes

Ingredients:

- 1 cup quinoa, rinsed
- 2 cups water or vegetable broth
- 2 cups broccoli florets, chopped
- 1 tablespoon olive oil
- 1 small onion, diced
- 2 cloves garlic, minced
- 4 large eggs
- 1/2 cup unsweetened almond milk
- 1/2 teaspoon salt
- 1/4 teaspoon black pepper
- 1/2 cup grated Parmesan cheese (optional for topping)

Nutritional Information: Estimated 300 calories, 15g protein, 35g carbohydrates, 12g fat, 5g fiber, 190mg cholesterol, 400mg sodium, 500mg potassium.

Directions:

1. Preheat the oven to 375°F (190°C). Bring the water or vegetable broth to a boil in a medium saucepan. Add the quinoa, reduce heat to low, cover, and simmer for 15 minutes or until all liquid is absorbed. Fluff with a fork and set aside.

2. While the quinoa cooks, heat the olive oil in a skillet over medium heat. Add the onion and garlic, sautéing until softened, about 3 minutes. Add the chopped broccoli and cook for an additional 5 minutes until the broccoli is just tender. Remove from heat.

3. Whisk the eggs, almond milk, salt, and pepper in a large mixing bowl. Stir in the cooked quinoa and broccoli mixture. Pour the mixture into a greased 9x9-inch baking dish. Sprinkle with grated Parmesan cheese if using.

4. Bake in the preheated oven for 25-30 minutes, or until the top is golden and a knife inserted into the center comes out clean. Let cool for a few minutes before serving.

Pumpkin Spice Chia Seed Pudding

Yield: 4 servings | **Prep time:** 10 minutes | **Cook time:** 0 minutes (plus at least 4 hours for chilling)

Ingredients:

- 1/4 cup chia seeds
- 1 cup unsweetened almond milk
- 3/4 cup pumpkin puree (not pumpkin pie filling)
- 2 tablespoons pure maple syrup
- 1 teaspoon vanilla extract
- 1/2 teaspoon ground cinnamon
- 1/4 teaspoon ground ginger
- 1/8 teaspoon ground nutmeg
- 1/8 teaspoon ground cloves
- Optional toppings: a sprinkle of ground cinnamon, chopped nuts, or a dollop of coconut yogurt

Nutritional Information: Estimated 150 calories, 4g protein, 20g carbohydrates, 7g fat, 8g fiber, 0mg cholesterol, 30mg sodium, 250mg potassium.

Directions:

1. Whisk the almond milk, pumpkin puree, maple syrup, vanilla extract, cinnamon, ginger, nutmeg, and cloves in a mixing bowl until smooth.
2. Stir in the chia seeds until well combined. Let the mixture sit for 5 minutes, then stir again to prevent the chia seeds from clumping.
3. Cover the bowl with plastic wrap or divide the mixture into individual serving containers. Refrigerate for at least 4 hours, or overnight, until the pudding has thickened and the chia seeds have fully absorbed the liquid.
4. Before serving, give the pudding a good stir. Adjust sweetness if necessary, and add more almond milk if the pudding is too thick. Serve with optional toppings, such as a sprinkle of cinnamon, chopped nuts, or a dollop of coconut yogurt.

Savory Turmeric and Black Pepper Oats with Avocado

Yield: 2 servings | **Prep time:** 5 minutes | **Cook time:** 10 minutes

Ingredients:

- 1 cup rolled oats (can be replaced with gluten-free oatmeal)
- 2 cups water or low-sodium vegetable broth
- 1/2 teaspoon ground turmeric
- 1/4 teaspoon ground black pepper
- 1/2 avocado, sliced
- 2 tablespoons chopped fresh cilantro
- 1 tablespoon lemon juice
- Salt to taste
- Optional: 2 tablespoons pumpkin seeds for garnish

Nutritional Information: Estimated 250 calories, 7g protein, 38g carbohydrates, 10g fat, 9g fiber, 0mg cholesterol, 30mg sodium, 300mg potassium.

Directions:

1. Bring the water or vegetable broth to a boil in a medium saucepan. Stir in the oats, turmeric, black pepper, and a pinch of salt. Reduce heat to a simmer and cook, stirring occasionally, until the oats are tender and have absorbed most of the liquid, about 5 to 7 minutes.
2. Remove from heat and let sit for a few minutes to thicken further.
3. Divide the cooked oats between two bowls. Top each serving with half of the sliced avocado and sprinkle with chopped cilantro. Drizzle with lemon juice and add pumpkin seeds for a crunchy garnish if desired.
4. Adjust salt to taste before serving.

Zucchini Bread with Flaxseeds

Yield: 6 servings | **Prep time:** 15 minutes | **Cook time:** 50 minutes

Ingredients:

- 1 1/2 cups whole wheat flour (can be replaced with any gluten-free flour)
- 1/2 cup ground flaxseeds
- 3/4 cup almond milk
- 2 teaspoons baking powder
- 1/2 teaspoon baking soda
- 1/2 teaspoon salt
- 1 teaspoon cinnamon
- 1/4 cup olive oil
- 1/2 cup maple syrup
- 1 teaspoon vanilla extract
- 2 cups grated zucchini (about 2 medium zucchini)
- Optional: 1/2 cup walnuts, chopped

Nutritional Information: Estimated 280 calories, 6g protein, 45g carbohydrates, 10g fat, 8g fiber, 0mg cholesterol, 320mg sodium, 200mg potassium.

Directions:

1. Preheat the oven to 350°F (175°C). Grease a 9x5 inch loaf pan or line it with parchment paper.
2. Whisk together the whole wheat flour, ground flaxseeds, baking powder, baking soda, salt, and cinnamon in a large bowl.
3. Mix the almond milk, olive oil, maple syrup, and vanilla extract in a separate bowl until well combined. Stir in the grated zucchini.
4. Add the wet ingredients to the dry ingredients, stirring just until combined. Fold in the walnuts if using.
5. Pour the batter into the prepared loaf pan. Bake for 50 minutes or until a toothpick inserted into the center comes clean.
6. Let the bread cool in the pan for 10 minutes, then transfer to a wire rack to cool completely before slicing.

Buckwheat Pancakes with Mixed Berry Compote

Yield: 4 servings | **Prep time:** 15 minutes | **Cook time:** 20 minutes

Ingredients:

For the Pancakes:

- 1 cup buckwheat flour
- 1 tablespoon baking powder
- 2 tablespoons pure maple syrup
- 1 cup unsweetened almond milk
- 1 egg
- 1 teaspoon vanilla extract
- Coconut oil for cooking

For the Mixed Berry Compote:

- 2 cups mixed berries (fresh or frozen)
- 2 tablespoons pure maple syrup
- 1/2 teaspoon lemon zest
- 1 tablespoon lemon juice

Nutritional Information: Estimated 280 calories, 8g protein, 50g carbohydrates, 5g fat, 7g fiber, 47mg cholesterol, 300mg sodium, 400mg potassium.

Directions:

1. Prepare the Mixed Berry Compote: In a small saucepan over medium heat, combine the mixed berries, maple syrup, lemon zest, and lemon juice. Simmer for 10-15 minutes, stirring occasionally, until the berries have softened and the sauce has thickened slightly. Remove from heat and set aside.
2. Make the Pancake Batter: Whisk together the buckwheat flour and baking powder in a large bowl. In a separate bowl, beat the egg and mix in the almond milk, maple syrup, and vanilla extract. Pour the wet ingredients into the dry ingredients, stirring until just combined.
3. Cook the Pancakes: Heat a skillet over medium heat and brush with a small amount of coconut oil. Pour 1/4 cup of batter for each pancake and cook for 2-3 minutes on each side until bubbles form on the surface and the edges look set. Flip and cook for an additional 2 minutes or until golden brown.
4. Serve: Divide the pancakes among plates and top with the warm mixed berry compote.

Anti-Inflammatory Breakfast Burritos

Yield: 4 servings | **Prep time:** 20 minutes | **Cook time:** 15 minutes

Ingredients:

- 4 whole grain or gluten-free tortillas
- 8 eggs
- 1 cup fresh spinach, chopped
- 1 medium avocado, sliced
- 1/2 cup black beans, rinsed and drained
- 1/2 cup cherry tomatoes, quartered
- 1/4 cup red onion, finely chopped
- 1 teaspoon olive oil
- 1/2 teaspoon turmeric
- 1/4 teaspoon garlic powder
- Salt and pepper to taste
- Optional: fresh cilantro and a squeeze of lime for garnish

Nutritional Information: Estimated 350 calories, 20g protein, 35g carbohydrates, 15g fat, 8g fiber, 372mg cholesterol, 400mg sodium, 600mg potassium.

Directions:

1. Heat the olive oil in a large skillet over medium heat. Add the red onion and sauté until translucent. Add the spinach and cook until just wilted. Remove from skillet and set aside.
2. In a bowl, whisk the eggs with turmeric, garlic powder, salt, and pepper. Pour the egg mixture into the same skillet and scramble over medium heat until cooked.
3. Warm the tortillas in a dry skillet or microwave for a few seconds until pliable.
4. Assemble the burritos: Lay out the tortillas and evenly distribute the scrambled eggs, sautéed spinach and onions, black beans, avocado slices, and cherry tomatoes among each tortilla. If desired, garnish with fresh cilantro and a squeeze of lime.
5. Roll up the tortillas, folding in the sides to enclose the filling. Serve immediately.

Kale, Pine Nut, and Raisin Morning Sauté

Yield: 4 servings | **Prep time:** 10 minutes | **Cook time:** 8 minutes

Ingredients:

- 4 cups kale, stems removed and leaves chopped
- 1/4 cup pine nuts
- 1/4 cup raisins
- 2 tablespoons olive oil
- 2 cloves garlic, minced
- Salt and pepper to taste
- Optional: 4 large eggs (if desired, for adding protein to the meal)

Nutritional Information: Estimated 200 calories, 5g protein (without eggs), 18g carbohydrates, 14g fat, 3g fiber, 0mg cholesterol (without eggs), 150mg sodium, 350mg potassium.

Directions:

1. Heat a large skillet over medium heat and add the pine nuts. Toast them, stirring frequently, until golden and fragrant, about 2-3 minutes. Remove from the skillet and set aside.
2. In the same skillet, heat the olive oil over medium heat. Add the minced garlic and sauté for about 1 minute until fragrant but not browned.
3. Add the chopped kale to the skillet, season with salt and pepper, and sauté for about 5 minutes, or until the kale has wilted and become tender. Add a tablespoon of water to help steam and wilt the kale if the kale sticks.
4. Stir in the raisins and toasted pine nuts, and cook for 2 minutes, allowing the flavors to meld together.
5. (Optional) In a separate pan, fry or poach eggs to your liking and serve on top of the kale mixture for added protein.

Mango and Turmeric Smoothie Bowl

Yield: 2 servings | **Prep time:** 10 minutes | **Cook time:** 0 minutes

Ingredients:

- 2 cups frozen mango chunks
- 1 banana, sliced
- 1/2 cup unsweetened almond milk
- 1 teaspoon ground turmeric
- 1/2 teaspoon ground ginger
- 1 tablespoon chia seeds
- Optional toppings: sliced almonds, fresh berries, coconut flakes, additional chia seeds

Nutritional Information: Estimated 250 calories, 4g protein, 50g carbohydrates, 5g fat, 7g fiber, 0mg cholesterol, 30mg sodium, 500mg potassium.

Directions:

1. Combine the frozen mango chunks, sliced banana, almond milk, ground turmeric, ginger, and chia seeds in a blender. Blend on high until smooth and creamy. Adjust the consistency by adding more almond milk if needed.
2. Pour the smoothie mixture into two bowls. Use the back of a spoon or spatula to spread the smoothie evenly.
3. Garnish each bowl with optional toppings: sliced almonds for crunch, fresh berries for extra antioxidants, coconut flakes for healthy fats, and additional chia seeds for fiber.
4. Serve immediately and enjoy this anti-inflammatory smoothie bowl's vibrant flavors and health benefits.

Egg White, Spinach, and Mushroom Breakfast Wraps

Yield: 4 servings | **Prep time:** 10 minutes | **Cook time:** 15 minutes

Ingredients:

- 8 large egg whites
- 2 cups fresh spinach, roughly chopped
- 1 cup mushrooms, sliced
- 1/4 cup red onion, finely diced
- 1 teaspoon olive oil
- 4 whole grain or gluten-free tortillas
- Salt and pepper to taste
- Optional: avocado slices or low-sodium salsa for serving

Nutritional Information: Estimated 200 calories, 18g protein, 25g carbohydrates, 5g fat, 4g fiber, 0mg cholesterol, 300mg sodium, 400mg potassium.

Directions:

1. Heat the olive oil in a large, non-stick skillet over medium heat. Add the mushrooms and red onion, sautéing until the vegetables are soft and slightly browned, about 5 minutes. Season with a bit of salt and pepper.
2. Add the chopped spinach to the skillet, cooking until it wilts, about 2-3 minutes. Remove the vegetables from the skillet and set aside.
3. In the same skillet, pour in the egg whites. Cook for about 2 minutes without stirring, then scramble until fully cooked, about 3 more minutes. Season with salt and pepper.
4. Warm the whole-grain tortillas according to package instructions. Divide the vegetable mixture and scrambled egg whites evenly among the tortillas. Add avocado slices or a spoonful of salsa on top of the eggs before rolling up the tortillas.
5. Roll up the tortillas, folding in the sides to enclose the filling, and serve immediately.

Savory Lentil and Sweet Potato Breakfast Bowl

Yield: 4 servings | **Prep time**: 15 minutes | **Cook time:** 30 minutes

Ingredients:

- 1 cup dried green lentils, rinsed
- 2 medium sweet potatoes, peeled and diced
- 1 tablespoon olive oil
- 1 teaspoon ground cumin
- 1/2 teaspoon smoked paprika
- Salt and pepper to taste
- 4 cups baby spinach
- Optional for serving: avocado slices, fresh cilantro, a drizzle of tahini

Nutritional Information: Estimated 350 calories, 18g protein, 55g carbohydrates, 5g fat, 15g fiber, 0mg cholesterol, 300mg sodium, 1000mg potassium.

Directions:

1. In a medium saucepan, bring 2 cups of water to a boil. Add the lentils, reduce heat to low, cover, and simmer for 20-25 minutes, or until lentils are tender but not mushy. Drain any excess water and set aside.
2. While the lentils are cooking, preheat the oven to 400°F (200°C). Toss the diced sweet potatoes with olive oil, ground cumin, smoked paprika, salt, and pepper. Spread in a single layer on a baking sheet and roast for 20-25 minutes or until tender and slightly caramelized, stirring halfway through.
3. In the last few minutes of cooking, wilt the spinach in a pan over medium heat with a splash of water, seasoning with a bit of salt and pepper.
4. To assemble the breakfast bowls, divide the cooked lentils, roasted sweet potatoes, and wilted spinach among four bowls. If desired, top with avocado slices, fresh cilantro, and a drizzle of tahini before serving.

Whole Grain Toast with Avocado and Sprouts

Yield: 2 servings | **Prep time:** 5 minutes | **Cook time:** 2 minutes

Ingredients:

- 2 slices of whole grain or gluten-free bread
- 1 ripe avocado
- 1/2 cup alfalfa sprouts
- 1 teaspoon lemon juice
- Salt and pepper to taste
- Optional toppings: radish slices, pumpkin seeds, or a drizzle of extra virgin olive oil

Nutritional Information: Estimated 250 calories, 8g protein, 30g carbohydrates, 14g fat, 10g fiber, 0mg cholesterol, 200mg sodium, 600mg potassium.

Directions:

1. Toast the whole grain bread slices to your desired level of crispness.
2. In a small bowl, mash the avocado with the lemon juice, salt, and pepper until it reaches a smooth consistency.
3. Spread the mashed avocado evenly over each slice of toasted bread.
4. Top each slice with a generous amount of alfalfa sprouts. If desired, add additional toppings like radish slices for crunch, pumpkin seeds for texture, or a drizzle of olive oil for extra flavor.
5. Serve immediately and enjoy a nutritious and satisfying breakfast or snack.

Spinach and Mushroom Egg Muffins

Yield: 6 servings | **Prep time:** 15 minutes | **Cook time:** 20 minutes

Ingredients:

- 10 large eggs
- 2 cups fresh spinach, roughly chopped
- 1 cup mushrooms, finely chopped
- 1/2 cup red bell pepper, diced
- 1/4 cup green onions, sliced
- Salt and pepper to taste
- Olive oil or cooking spray for greasing

Nutritional Information: Estimated 150 calories, 13g protein, 3g carbohydrates, 10g fat, 1g fiber, 310mg cholesterol, 125mg sodium, 200mg potassium per serving.

Directions:

1. Preheat your oven to 350°F (175°C). Grease a 12-slot muffin pan with olive oil or cooking spray.
2. In a large mixing bowl, beat the eggs until smooth. Season with salt and pepper.
3. Stir in the spinach, mushrooms, red bell pepper, and green onions until well combined.
4. Pour the egg mixture evenly into the prepared muffin pan slots, filling each about two-thirds full.
5. Bake in the preheated oven for 18-20 minutes or until the egg muffins are firm and lightly golden on top.
6. Allow it to cool for a few minutes before removing it from the pan. Serve warm.

Avocado Berry Smoothie Bowl

Yield: 2 servings | **Prep time:** 10 minutes | **Cook time:** 0 minutes

Ingredients:

- 1 ripe avocado, halved and pitted
- 1 cup frozen mixed berries (such as strawberries, blueberries, and raspberries)
- 1 banana, sliced
- 1/2 cup unsweetened almond milk
- 1 tablespoon chia seeds
- Optional toppings: sliced almonds, coconut flakes, fresh berries, hemp seeds

Nutritional Information: Estimated 300 calories, 6g protein, 35g carbohydrates, 18g fat, 10g fiber, 0mg cholesterol, 70mg sodium, 600mg potassium.

Directions:

1. Scoop the avocado flesh into a blender. Add the frozen mixed berries, banana, almond milk, and chia seeds.
2. Blend on high until smooth and creamy. Adjust the consistency by adding more almond milk if needed.
3. Pour the smoothie mixture into two bowls.
4. Garnish each bowl with toppings: sliced almonds for crunch, coconut flakes for sweetness, fresh berries for antioxidants, and hemp seeds for additional protein and omega-3 fatty acids.
5. Serve immediately and enjoy a nutritious, anti-inflammatory breakfast.

Sweet Potato Toast with Avocado Mash

Yield: 4 servings | **Prep time:** 10 minutes | **Cook time:** 15 minutes

Ingredients:

- 2 large sweet potatoes, sliced lengthwise into 1/4-inch thick slices
- 2 ripe avocados
- Juice of 1 lime
- Salt and pepper to taste
- Optional toppings: cherry tomatoes (halved), radish slices, crushed red pepper flakes, or cilantro

Nutritional Information: Estimated 250 calories, 4g protein, 30g carbohydrates, 15g fat, 7g fiber, 0mg cholesterol, 30mg sodium, 800mg potassium.

Directions:

1. Preheat your toaster oven or conventional oven to 400°F (200°C). If using a traditional oven, place the sweet potato slices on a baking sheet lined with parchment paper.
2. Toast or bake the sweet potato slices for 15 minutes, flipping halfway through or until they are tender and slightly crispy on the edges.
3. While the sweet potatoes are toasting, mash the avocados in a bowl with lime juice, salt, and pepper until you reach your desired consistency.
4. Once the sweet potato slices are done, allow them to cool for a minute. Then, spread a generous layer of avocado mash on each slice.
5. For extra flavor and nutrition, top with optional toppings such as cherry tomatoes, radish slices, crushed red pepper flakes, or cilantro.
6. Serve immediately and enjoy a nutritious, anti-inflammatory breakfast or snack.

Kale and Quinoa Breakfast Salad

Yield: 4 servings | **Prep time:** 15 minutes | **Cook time:** 20 minutes

Ingredients:

- 1 cup quinoa, rinsed
- 2 cups water
- 4 cups kale, stems removed and leaves chopped
- 1 tablespoon olive oil
- 2 tablespoons lemon juice
- 1 avocado, diced
- 1/4 cup almonds, sliced and toasted
- Salt and pepper to taste
- Optional: 4 eggs (for topping)

Nutritional Information: Estimated 300 calories, 10g protein, 35g carbohydrates, 15g fat, 8g fiber, 0mg cholesterol (without eggs), 200mg sodium, 600mg potassium.

Directions:

1. In a medium saucepan, bring 2 cups of water to a boil. Add the quinoa, reduce the heat to low, cover it, and simmer it for about 15 minutes, or until the water is absorbed and the quinoa is tender. Fluff with a fork and set aside to cool slightly.
2. While the quinoa is cooking, massage the kale with olive oil in a large bowl until the leaves soften, about 2-3 minutes. Add the lemon juice and a pinch of salt and pepper, and toss to combine.
3. Add the cooked quinoa to the kale in the bowl. Toss well to combine. Gently fold in the diced avocado and toasted almonds.
4. (Optional) In a separate pan, cook the eggs to your liking (poached, fried, or boiled) and place one egg on each salad serving.
5. Serve the salad warm or at room temperature, with an optional egg on top for added protein.

Smoked Salmon and Avocado Wrap

Yield: 4 servings | **Prep time:** 15 minutes | **Cook time:** 0 minutes

Ingredients:

- 4 whole grain or gluten-free tortillas
- 8 ounces smoked salmon
- 2 ripe avocados, mashed
- 1 cup mixed greens (e.g., arugula, spinach)
- 1/2 cucumber, thinly sliced
- 1/4 red onion, thinly sliced
- 2 tablespoons capers, rinsed
- 1 tablespoon lemon juice
- Salt and pepper to taste
- Optional: 1 tablespoon dill, chopped

Nutritional Information: Estimated 350 calories, 23g protein, 37g carbohydrates, 15g fat, 7g fiber, 20mg cholesterol, 600mg sodium, 800mg potassium.

Directions:

1. Lay out the whole-grain tortillas on a flat surface. Spread the mashed avocado evenly across each tortilla, leaving a small border around the edges.
2. Drizzle lemon juice over the mashed avocado and season with salt and pepper.
3. Arrange the smoked salmon slices over the avocado. Top with mixed greens, cucumber slices, red onion, capers, and dill (if using).
4. Carefully roll up each tortilla, folding in the sides as you go, to enclose the filling. If necessary, secure the wraps with toothpicks.
5. Cut each wrap in half and serve immediately, or wrap them in parchment paper for an on-the-go breakfast or lunch.

Walnut and Pumpkin Seed Granola

Yield: 6 servings | **Prep time:** 10 minutes | **Cook time:** 20 minutes

Ingredients:

- 2 cups oats (can be replaced with gluten-free oatmeal)
- 1/2 cup walnuts, roughly chopped
- 1/2 cup pumpkin seeds (pepitas)
- 1/4 cup ground flaxseed
- 1/4 cup honey or maple syrup
- 1/4 cup coconut oil, melted
- 1 teaspoon vanilla extract
- 1/2 teaspoon ground cinnamon
- 1/4 teaspoon salt
- Optional: 1/2 cup dried unsweetened cranberries or cherries, added after baking

Nutritional Information: Estimated 300 calories, 8g protein, 28g carbohydrates, 18g fat, 5g fiber, 0mg cholesterol, 100mg sodium, 250mg potassium.

Directions:

1. Preheat your oven to 300°F (150°C). Line a baking sheet with parchment paper.
2. Mix the oats, walnuts, pumpkin seeds, and ground flaxseed in a large bowl.
3. In a separate small bowl, whisk together the honey (or maple syrup), melted coconut oil, vanilla extract, cinnamon, and salt until well combined.
4. Pour the wet ingredients over the dry ingredients and stir until evenly coated.
5. Spread the granola mixture in an even layer on the prepared baking sheet. Bake in the preheated oven for 20 minutes, stirring halfway through the cooking time, until the granola is golden brown and fragrant.
6. Let the granola cool completely on the baking sheet. If using, stir in the dried cranberries or cherries. Store the granola in an airtight container at room temperature for up to 2 weeks.

Zucchini and Carrot Pancakes

Yield: 4 servings | **Prep time:** 15 minutes | **Cook time:** 10 minutes

Ingredients:

- 1 medium zucchini, grated
- 2 medium carrots, grated
- 2 large eggs
- 1/2 cup almond flour
- 1/4 cup green onions, finely chopped
- 1 garlic clove, minced
- 1/2 teaspoon salt
- 1/4 teaspoon ground black pepper
- 2 tablespoons olive oil for frying

Nutritional Information: Estimated 220 calories, 8g protein, 12g carbohydrates, 16g fat, 3g fiber, 93mg cholesterol, 320mg sodium, 400mg potassium per serving.

Directions:

1. Place the grated zucchini and carrots in a clean kitchen towel and squeeze out as much liquid as possible.
2. Combine the squeezed zucchini and carrots, eggs, almond flour, green onions, minced garlic, salt, and pepper in a large bowl. Stir until well mixed.
3. Heat olive oil in a large skillet over medium heat. Scoop 1/4 cup portions of the zucchini and carrot mixture into the skillet, flattening them slightly with the back of the scoop to form pancakes.
4. Cook for 3-5 minutes on each side until golden brown is cooked through. Transfer to a paper towel-lined plate to drain any excess oil.
5. Serve warm, optionally, with plain Greek yogurt or your favorite sauce.

Buckwheat and Blueberry Porridge

Yield: 4 servings | **Prep time:** 5 minutes | **Cook time:** 15 minutes

Ingredients:

- 1 cup buckwheat groats
- 3 cups unsweetened almond milk
- 1 cup fresh or frozen blueberries
- 2 tablespoons maple syrup or honey
- 1 teaspoon vanilla extract
- 1/2 teaspoon ground cinnamon
- Pinch of salt
- Optional toppings: additional blueberries, sliced almonds, chia seeds

Nutritional Information: Estimated 220 calories, 6g protein, 40g carbohydrates, 3g fat, 6g fiber, 0mg cholesterol, 80mg sodium, 300mg potassium per serving.

Directions:

1. Rinse the buckwheat groats under cold water until the water runs clear.
2. Bring the almond milk to a simmer over medium heat in a medium saucepan. Add the rinsed buckwheat groats, maple syrup (or honey), vanilla extract, ground cinnamon, and a pinch of salt. Stir to combine.
3. Reduce the heat to low and simmer, covered, for 10-15 minutes, or until the buckwheat is tender and most of the liquid has been absorbed. Stir occasionally to prevent sticking, adding more almond milk if needed for your desired consistency.
4. Once the porridge is cooked, gently fold in the blueberries, allowing them to heat through for about 1-2 minutes, especially if using frozen blueberries.
5. Serve the porridge hot with optional toppings like additional blueberries, sliced almonds, or chia seeds sprinkled on top.

Cinnamon Apple Quinoa Breakfast Bowl

Yield: 4 servings | **Prep time:** 10 minutes | **Cook time:** 20 minutes

Ingredients:

- 1 cup quinoa, rinsed
- 2 cups water
- 2 apples, diced
- 1 teaspoon ground cinnamon
- 1/4 teaspoon nutmeg
- 2 tablespoons maple syrup
- 1/2 cup unsweetened almond milk
- Optional toppings: chopped nuts (walnuts, almonds), fresh berries, additional maple syrup

Nutritional Information: Estimated 220 calories, 6g protein, 45g carbohydrates, 3g fat, 5g fiber, 0mg cholesterol, 30mg sodium, 400mg potassium per serving.

Directions:

1. Combine quinoa and water in a medium saucepan. Bring to a boil, then reduce heat to low, cover, and simmer for 15 minutes, until quinoa is cooked and water is absorbed. Fluff with a fork and set aside.
2. While the quinoa is cooking, add the diced apples, cinnamon, nutmeg, and maple syrup to a separate saucepan. Cook over medium heat for about 5-7 minutes or until the apples are soft and the mixture is fragrant.
3. Stir the cooked apples and almond milk into the cooked quinoa, mixing until well combined. Heat through for 2-3 minutes, adding more almond milk if a creamier consistency is desired.
4. Serve the quinoa and apple mixture in bowls, topped with chopped nuts, fresh berries, or an extra drizzle of maple syrup.

Poached Eggs over Spinach and Arugula Greens

Yield: 4 servings | **Prep time:** 10 minutes | **Cook time:** 10 minutes

Ingredients:

- Four large eggs
- 4 cups baby spinach leaves
- 4 cups arugula leaves
- 2 teaspoons olive oil
- 1 garlic clove, minced
- Salt and pepper to taste
- Optional garnish: shaved Parmesan cheese, red pepper flakes

Nutritional Information: Estimated 150 calories, 10g protein, 3g carbohydrates, 11g fat, 2g fiber, 186mg cholesterol, 200mg sodium, 300mg potassium per serving.

Directions:

1. Heat the olive oil in a large skillet over medium heat. Add the minced garlic and sauté for about 1 minute until fragrant but not browned. Add the spinach and arugula leaves, seasoning with salt and pepper. Cook, stirring occasionally, until the greens are wilted, about 3-5 minutes. Remove from heat and divide the greens evenly among four plates.

2. Fill a large saucepan with about 3 inches of water and bring to a simmer. Add a pinch of salt. Crack each egg into a small bowl and gently slide it into the simmering water. Cook for about 4 minutes for soft yolks or longer for firmer yolks. A slotted spoon removes the eggs from the water, draining well.

3. Place a poached egg on top of the greens on each plate. Season with salt and pepper to taste.

4. Garnish with shaved Parmesan cheese and a sprinkle of red pepper flakes before serving.

Lunch

Quinoa Salad with Chickpeas and Avocado

Yield: 4 servings | **Prep time:** 15 minutes | **Cook time:** 15 minutes

Ingredients:

- 1 cup quinoa
- 2 cups water
- 1 can (15 ounces) chickpeas, drained and rinsed
- 1 large avocado, diced
- 1 cup cherry tomatoes, halved
- 1/2 cucumber, diced
- 1/4 cup red onion, finely chopped
- 1/4 cup fresh parsley, chopped
- 2 tablespoons olive oil
- Juice of 1 lemon
- Salt and pepper to taste

Nutritional Information: Estimated 320 calories, 10g protein, 45g carbohydrates, 12g fat, 8g fiber, 0mg cholesterol, 200mg sodium, 600mg potassium per serving.

Directions:

1. Rinse quinoa under cold water. In a medium saucepan, bring 2 cups of water to a boil. Add quinoa, reduce heat to low, cover, and simmer for about 15 minutes, until all water is absorbed and quinoa is fluffy. Allow to cool.
2. Combine cooled quinoa, chickpeas, avocado, cherry tomatoes, cucumber, red onion, and parsley in a large bowl.
3. Whisk together olive oil, lemon juice, salt, and pepper in a small bowl. Pour dressing over the quinoa mixture and toss gently to combine.
4. Taste and adjust seasoning as needed. Serve immediately or refrigerate until ready to serve.

Grilled Chicken and Roasted Vegetable Bowl

Yield: 4 servings | **Prep time:** 20 minutes | **Cook time:** 30 minutes

Ingredients:

- 2 large chicken breasts, boneless and skinless
- 1 tablespoon olive oil (for chicken)
- 1 teaspoon garlic powder
- Salt and pepper to taste
- 2 cups broccoli florets
- 1 red bell pepper, sliced
- 1 zucchini, sliced
- 1 sweet potato, peeled and cubed
- 2 tablespoons olive oil (for vegetables)
- 1/2 teaspoon smoked paprika
- 1 cup cooked quinoa
- Optional: lemon wedges and fresh parsley for garnish

Nutritional Information: Estimated 400 calories, 30g protein, 40g carbohydrates, 15g fat, 8g fiber, 75mg cholesterol, 300mg sodium, 800mg potassium per serving.

Directions:

1. Preheat your grill to medium-high heat and preheat the oven to 425°F (220°C). Toss the broccoli, bell pepper, zucchini, and sweet potato with 2 tablespoons of olive oil, smoked paprika, salt, and pepper. Spread the vegetables on a baking sheet and roast for 25-30 minutes or until tender and slightly caramelized, stirring halfway through.
2. While the vegetables are roasting, rub the chicken breasts with 1 tablespoon of olive oil, garlic powder, salt, and pepper. Grill the chicken for 6-7 minutes per side or until fully cooked through, and the internal temperature reaches 165°F (74°C). Let it rest for a few minutes, then slice thinly.
3. Divide the cooked quinoa among bowls. Top with a mix of roasted vegetables and sliced grilled chicken.
4. Garnish with lemon wedges and fresh parsley if desired before serving.

Lentil Soup with Kale and Sweet Potatoes

Yield: 4 servings | **Prep time:** 15 minutes | **Cook time:** 40 minutes

Ingredients:

- 1 cup dry green lentils, rinsed
- 1 large sweet potato, peeled and cubed
- 2 cups kale, stems removed and leaves chopped
- 1 large onion, diced
- 2 cloves garlic, minced
- 2 carrots, peeled and diced
- 2 stalks celery, diced
- 4 cups vegetable broth
- 2 cups water
- 2 tablespoons olive oil
- 1 teaspoon ground cumin
- 1/2 teaspoon smoked paprika
- Salt and pepper to taste
- Optional: fresh lemon juice for serving

Nutritional Information: Estimated 300 calories, 18g protein, 55g carbohydrates, 5g fat, 15g fiber, 0mg cholesterol, 300mg sodium, 800mg potassium per serving.

Directions:

1. Heat olive oil in a large pot over medium heat. Add the onion, garlic, carrots, celery, and sauté for about 5 minutes until the vegetables are softened.
2. Stir in the ground cumin and smoked paprika, cooking for another minute until fragrant.
3. Add the rinsed lentils, cubed sweet potato, vegetable broth, and water to the pot. Bring to a boil, then reduce the heat to low, cover, and simmer for 25-30 minutes or until the lentils and sweet potatoes are tender.
4. Stir in the chopped kale and continue to simmer for another 5-10 minutes until the kale is wilted and tender. Season the soup with salt and pepper to taste.
5. Serve the soup hot, with a squeeze of fresh lemon juice if desired.

Turmeric-Spiced Salmon with Brown Rice

Yield: 4 servings | **Prep time:** 10 minutes | **Cook time:** 30 minutes

Ingredients:

- 4 salmon fillets (6 ounces each)
- 1 cup brown rice
- 2 cups water
- 2 tablespoons olive oil
- 1 teaspoon ground turmeric
- 1/2 teaspoon garlic powder
- 1/2 teaspoon ground ginger
- Salt and pepper to taste
- Optional: lemon wedges and fresh parsley for garnish

Nutritional Information: Estimated 400 calories, 34g protein, 38g carbohydrates, 14g fat, 3g fiber, 75mg cholesterol, 200mg sodium, 800mg potassium per serving.

Directions:

1. Rinse the brown rice under cold water. In a medium saucepan, bring 2 cups of water to a boil. Add the brown rice, reduce the heat to low, cover, and simmer for about 25-30 minutes, or until the water is absorbed and the rice is tender.
2. While the rice is cooking, preheat the oven to 375°F (190°C). Line a baking sheet with parchment paper.
3. Mix the olive oil, turmeric, garlic powder, ground ginger, salt, and pepper in a small bowl. Brush this mixture over both sides of the salmon fillets.
4. Place the salmon on the prepared baking sheet and bake for 12-15 minutes or until the salmon is flaky and cooked.
5. Serve the salmon over a bed of brown rice. Garnish with lemon wedges and fresh parsley if desired.

Vegan Black Bean and Quinoa Stuffed Peppers

Yield: 4 servings | **Prep time:** 15 minutes | **Cook time:** 40 minutes

Ingredients:

- 4 large bell peppers, halved and seeds removed
- 1 cup quinoa, rinsed
- 2 cups vegetable broth
- 1 can (15 ounces) black beans, drained and rinsed
- 1 cup corn kernels (fresh or frozen)
- 1/2 cup red onion, finely chopped
- 1 teaspoon ground cumin
- 1/2 teaspoon chili powder
- Salt and pepper to taste
- 1/4 cup fresh cilantro, chopped
- Optional: avocado slices, lime wedges, and salsa for serving

Nutritional Information: Estimated 250 calories, 10g protein, 45g carbohydrates, 3g fat, 10g fiber, 0mg cholesterol, 300mg sodium, 700mg potassium per serving.

Directions:

1. Preheat the oven to 375°F (190°C). Arrange the bell pepper halves in a baking dish, cut side up.
2. In a medium saucepan, bring the vegetable broth to a boil. Add the quinoa, reduce the heat to low, cover it, and simmer it for about 15 minutes until all the broth is absorbed and the quinoa is tender. Fluff with a fork and set aside.
3. In a large bowl, combine the cooked quinoa, black beans, corn, red onion, cumin, chili powder, salt, pepper, and cilantro. Mix well to combine.
4. Spoon the quinoa and bean mixture into each bell pepper half, pressing down slightly to pack the filling.
5. Cover the baking dish with aluminum foil and bake for about 25 minutes. Remove the foil and bake for 15 minutes until the peppers are tender and the filling is heated through.
6. Serve the stuffed peppers with optional avocado slices, lime wedges, and salsa on the side.

Baked Tofu and Vegetable Stir-Fry over Whole Grain Noodles

Yield: 4 servings | **Prep time:** 20 minutes | **Cook time:** 30 minutes

Ingredients:

- 14 ounces extra-firm tofu, pressed and cubed
- 2 tablespoons soy sauce (or tamari for gluten-free)
- 1 tablespoon sesame oil
- 1 tablespoon maple syrup
- 2 cups broccoli florets
- 1 red bell pepper, sliced
- 1 carrot, julienned
- 1 cup snap peas
- 8 ounces whole grain (or gluten-free) noodles
- 2 cloves garlic, minced
- 1-inch ginger, grated
- 2 tablespoons olive oil
- Optional garnishes: sesame seeds, sliced green onions

Nutritional Information: Estimated 450 calories, 20g protein, 65g carbohydrates, 15g fat, 10g fiber, 0mg cholesterol, 400mg sodium, 500mg potassium per serving.

Directions:

1. Preheat the oven to 400°F (200°C). Toss the cubed tofu with soy sauce, sesame oil, and maple syrup. Spread in a single layer on a baking sheet lined with parchment paper. Bake for 25-30 minutes or until crispy, turning halfway through.
2. Cook the whole grain noodles according to package instructions, drain, and set aside.
3. Heat the olive oil over medium-high heat in a large skillet or wok. Add the garlic and ginger, sautéing for about 1 minute until fragrant. Add the broccoli, bell pepper, carrot, and snap peas. Stir-fry for 5-7 minutes or until vegetables are tender but crisp.
4. Add the baked tofu and cooked noodles to the skillet with the vegetables. Toss everything together, heating through. Adjust seasoning with additional soy sauce if needed.
5. Serve the stir-fry in bowls, garnished with sesame seeds and sliced green onions if desired.

Spicy Sweet Potato and Black Bean Burrito Bowl

Yield: 4 servings | **Prep time:** 15 minutes | **Cook time:** 30 minutes

Ingredients:

- 2 large sweet potatoes, peeled and cubed
- 1 tablespoon olive oil
- 1 teaspoon chili powder
- 1/2 teaspoon cumin
- Salt and pepper to taste
- 1 can (15 ounces) black beans, drained and rinsed
- 2 cups cooked brown rice
- 1 avocado, sliced
- 1 cup cherry tomatoes, halved
- 1/4 cup red onion, finely chopped
- 1 lime, juiced
- 1/4 cup fresh cilantro, chopped
- Optional: jalapeño slices, Greek yogurt, or salsa for topping

Nutritional Information: Estimated 400 calories, 12g protein, 60g carbohydrates, 12g fat, 12g fiber, 0mg cholesterol, 300mg sodium, 800mg potassium per serving.

Directions:

1. Preheat the oven to 425°F (220°C). Toss the cubed sweet potatoes with olive oil, chili powder, cumin, salt, and pepper on a baking sheet. Roast in the preheated oven for 25-30 minutes or until tender and lightly caramelized, stirring halfway through.
2. While the sweet potatoes are roasting, prepare the brown rice according to package instructions.
3. Mix the black beans in a bowl with half of the lime juice and a pinch of salt. Warm them up if desired.
4. Assemble the burrito bowls by dividing the cooked brown rice among four bowls. Top each with roasted sweet potatoes, black beans, avocado slices, cherry tomatoes, and red onion.
5. Drizzle the remaining lime juice over each bowl and garnish with fresh cilantro. Add optional toppings like jalapeño slices, Greek yogurt, or salsa to taste.

Grilled Vegetable and Hummus Wraps

Yield: 4 servings | **Prep time:** 15 minutes | **Cook time:** 10 minutes

Ingredients:

- 2 zucchinis, sliced lengthwise
- 2 red bell peppers, seeded and quartered
- 1 eggplant, sliced into rounds
- 2 tablespoons olive oil
- Salt and pepper to taste
- 4 large whole-grain (or gluten-free) tortillas
- 1 cup hummus
- 2 cups mixed greens (such as arugula and spinach)
- Optional: feta cheese, sun-dried tomatoes, or olives for added flavor

Nutritional Information: Estimated 350 calories, 12g protein, 45g carbohydrates, 15g fat, 10g fiber, 0mg cholesterol, 400mg sodium, 600mg potassium per serving.

Directions:

1. Preheat a grill or grill pan over medium-high heat. Brush the zucchini, bell peppers, and eggplant slices with olive oil and season with salt and pepper.
2. Grill the vegetables in batches, turning once, until they are tender and have grill marks, about 3-5 minutes per side. Remove from the grill and set aside.
3. Warm the whole grain tortillas on the grill for about 30 seconds on each side until they are pliable.
4. Spread a generous layer of hummus over each tortilla. Layer the grilled vegetables and mixed greens on one end of each tortilla. If using, add feta cheese, sun-dried tomatoes, or olives.
5. Roll up the tortillas tightly, folding in the sides as you roll, to enclose the filling. Cut each wrap in half and serve immediately.

Cauliflower Rice Tabbouleh with Grilled Chicken

Yield: 4 servings | **Prep time:** 20 minutes | **Cook time:** 20 minutes

Ingredients:

- 2 large chicken breasts
- Salt and pepper to taste
- 1 tablespoon olive oil (for chicken)
- 1 head of cauliflower, riced
- 1 large cucumber, diced
- 2 medium tomatoes, diced
- 1/4 cup red onion, finely chopped
- 1 cup fresh parsley, chopped
- 1/2 cup fresh mint, chopped
- 3 tablespoons olive oil (for tabbouleh)
- Juice of 2 lemons
- Optional: lemon wedges for serving

Nutritional Information: Estimated 300 calories, 25g protein, 18g carbohydrates, 15g fat, 6g fiber, 65mg cholesterol, 200mg sodium, 800mg potassium per serving.

Directions:

1. Preheat the grill to medium-high heat. Season the chicken breasts with salt, pepper, and 1 tablespoon olive oil. Grill for 10 minutes on each side or until the internal temperature reaches 165°F (74°C). Let the chicken rest for a few minutes before slicing thinly.
2. To prepare the cauliflower rice, pulse cauliflower florets in a food processor until it resembles rice. You can also use pre-riced cauliflower to save time.
3. Combine the riced cauliflower, diced cucumber, tomatoes, red onion, parsley, and mint in a large bowl. Toss with 3 tablespoons of olive oil and the lemon juice. Season with salt and pepper to taste.
4. Divide the cauliflower rice tabbouleh among serving plates. Top with sliced grilled chicken. Serve with lemon wedges on the side if desired.

Spinach, Walnut, and Strawberry Salad with Grilled Shrimp

Yield: 4 servings | **Prep time:** 15 minutes | **Cook time:** 10 minutes

Ingredients:

- 1 pound large shrimp, peeled and deveined
- 1 tablespoon olive oil (for shrimp)
- Salt and pepper to taste
- 8 cups fresh baby spinach
- 1 cup strawberries, sliced
- 1/2 cup walnuts, toasted
- 1/4 cup feta cheese, crumbled
- 2 tablespoons balsamic vinegar
- 1 tablespoon honey
- 3 tablespoons olive oil (for dressing)
- Optional: fresh basil leaves for garnish

Nutritional Information: Estimated 350 calories, 25g protein, 12g carbohydrates, 24g fat, 4g fiber, 180mg cholesterol, 300mg sodium, 500mg potassium per serving.

Directions:

1. Preheat the grill to medium-high heat. Toss the shrimp with 1 tablespoon of olive oil, salt, and pepper. Grill the shrimp on each side for 2-3 minutes until they are pink and opaque. Remove from the grill and set aside.
2. Combine the baby spinach, sliced strawberries, toasted walnuts, and crumbled feta cheese in a large salad bowl.
3. Whisk together the balsamic vinegar, honey, and 3 tablespoons of olive oil in a small bowl to create the dressing. Season with salt and pepper to taste.
4. Drizzle the dressing over the salad and toss gently to coat.
5. Divide the salad among serving plates and top with grilled shrimp. Garnish with fresh basil leaves if desired.

Zucchini Noodles with Avocado Pesto and Cherry Tomatoes

Yield: 4 servings | **Prep time:** 15 minutes | **Cook time:** 0 minutes

Ingredients:

- 4 medium zucchinis, spiralized into noodles
- 1 ripe avocado
- 1/2 cup fresh basil leaves
- 1/4 cup pine nuts
- 2 cloves garlic, minced
- 2 tablespoons lemon juice
- 1/4 cup olive oil
- Salt and pepper to taste
- 1 cup cherry tomatoes, halved
- Optional: red pepper flakes for extra spice

Nutritional Information: Estimated 250 calories, 4g protein, 15g carbohydrates, 20g fat, 6g fiber, 0mg cholesterol, 100mg sodium, 500mg potassium per serving.

Directions:

1. To make the avocado pesto, blend the avocado, basil leaves, pine nuts, garlic, and lemon juice in a food processor until smooth. With the processor running, slowly add the olive oil until the mixture is creamy. Season with salt and pepper to taste.
2. Place the spiralized zucchini noodles in a large bowl. Add the avocado pesto to the zucchini noodles and toss until well-coated.
3. Gently fold in the cherry tomatoes, being careful not to crush them. Season with additional salt and pepper if needed.
4. Divide the zucchini noodles among serving plates. If desired, sprinkle with red pepper flakes for a bit of heat.
5. Serve immediately, or chill in the refrigerator for a refreshing cold salad.

Moroccan Lentil and Vegetable Stew

Yield: 4 servings | **Prep time:** 15 minutes | **Cook time:** 45 minutes

Ingredients:

- 1 cup dry green lentils, rinsed
- 2 tablespoons olive oil
- 1 large onion, chopped
- 2 cloves garlic, minced
- 2 carrots, peeled and diced
- 2 celery stalks, diced
- 1 sweet potato, peeled and cubed
- 1 teaspoon ground cumin
- 1 teaspoon ground coriander
- 1/2 teaspoon ground cinnamon
- 1/4 teaspoon ground turmeric
- 1 can (14.5 ounces) diced tomatoes
- 4 cups vegetable broth
- Salt and pepper to taste
- 1 cup chopped kale or spinach
- Optional: chopped fresh cilantro and lemon wedges for serving

Nutritional Information: Estimated 300 calories, 18g protein, 55g carbohydrates, 5g fat, 15g fiber, 0mg cholesterol, 300mg sodium, 800mg potassium per serving.

Directions:

1. In a large pot, heat the olive oil over medium heat. Add the onion and garlic, sautéing until the onion is translucent, about 5 minutes.
2. Add the carrots, celery, and sweet potato to the pot. Cook for another 5 minutes, stirring occasionally.
3. Stir in the cumin, coriander, cinnamon, and turmeric, cooking until fragrant, about 1 minute. Add the lentils, diced tomatoes (with their juice), and vegetable broth. Season with salt and pepper.
4. Bring the mixture to a boil, then reduce the heat to low and simmer, covered, for about 30 minutes or until the lentils and vegetables are tender.
5. Stir in the kale or spinach and cook until wilted, about 5 minutes. Adjust seasoning as needed.
6. Serve hot, garnished with fresh cilantro and lemon wedges on the side if desired.

Beetroot, Goat Cheese, and Arugula Salad with Roasted Beets

Yield: 4 servings | **Prep time:** 10 minutes | **Cook time:** 40 minutes

Ingredients:

- 4 medium beetroots, scrubbed and trimmed
- 4 cups arugula leaves, washed
- 1/2 cup goat cheese, crumbled
- 1/4 cup walnuts, toasted and chopped
- 2 tablespoons balsamic vinegar
- 1/4 cup extra-virgin olive oil
- Salt and pepper to taste
- Optional: fresh thyme leaves or honey for garnish

Nutritional Information: Estimated 250 calories, 7g protein, 15g carbohydrates, 19g fat, 4g fiber, 13mg cholesterol, 200mg sodium, 500mg potassium per serving.

Directions:

1. Preheat the oven to 400°F (200°C). Wrap each beetroot in foil and place on a baking sheet. Roast in the preheated oven for 40 minutes or until tender when pierced with a fork. Once cool enough to handle, peel the beetroots and cut into wedges.
2. Combine the arugula leaves, roasted beet wedges, crumbled goat cheese, and toasted walnuts in a large salad bowl.
3. Whisk together the balsamic vinegar, olive oil, salt, and pepper in a small bowl to create the dressing.
4. Drizzle the dressing over the salad and gently toss to coat evenly.
5. Serve the salad garnished with fresh thyme leaves or a desired drizzle of honey.

Soba Noodles with Edamame and Cucumber

Yield: 4 servings | **Prep time:** 10 minutes | **Cook time:** 10 minutes

Ingredients:

- 8 ounces soba noodles (or gluten-free noodles)
- 1 cup edamame, shelled and cooked
- 1 large cucumber, julienned or spiralized
- 1/4 cup soy sauce (or tamari for a gluten-free option)
- 1 tablespoon sesame oil
- 2 tablespoons rice vinegar
- 1 teaspoon honey or maple syrup
- 1 clove garlic, minced
- 1-inch piece of ginger, grated
- Optional: sesame seeds and sliced green onions for garnish

Nutritional Information: Estimated 320 calories, 12g protein, 50g carbohydrates, 7g fat, 3g fiber, 0mg cholesterol, 620mg sodium, 400mg potassium per serving.

Directions:

- Cook the soba noodles according to package instructions, then rinse under cold water and drain.
- Mix the cooked soba noodles, edamame, and julienned cucumber in a large bowl.
- In a small bowl, whisk together the soy sauce, sesame oil, rice vinegar, honey (or maple syrup), minced garlic, and grated ginger to create the dressing.
- Pour the dressing over the noodle mixture and toss to combine thoroughly.
- Serve the noodles chilled or at room temperature, garnished with sesame seeds and sliced green onions if desired.

Spiced Chickpea and Roasted Cauliflower Pita Pockets

Yield: 4 servings | **Prep time:** 15 minutes | **Cook time:** 25 minutes

Ingredients:

- 1 can (15 ounces) chickpeas, drained and rinsed
- 1 small head cauliflower, cut into florets
- 2 tablespoons olive oil, divided
- 1 teaspoon ground cumin
- 1/2 teaspoon smoked paprika
- Salt and pepper to taste
- 4 whole grain pita bread (or gluten-free)
- 1 cup spinach leaves
- 1/2 cucumber, thinly sliced
- 1/4 cup plain Greek yogurt (or plant-based)
- 1 tablespoon lemon juice
- 1 garlic clove, minced
- Optional: fresh cilantro or parsley for garnish

Nutritional Information: Estimated 350 calories, 12g protein, 55g carbohydrates, 9g fat, 10g fiber, 5mg cholesterol, 400mg sodium, 700mg potassium per serving.

Directions:

1. Preheat the oven to 425°F (220°C). Toss the cauliflower florets with 1 tablespoon of olive oil, cumin, smoked paprika, salt, and pepper. Spread on a baking sheet and roast for 20-25 minutes or until tender and golden.
2. Mix the chickpeas with the remaining 1 tablespoon of olive oil, a pinch of salt, and pepper in a bowl. Spread them on a separate baking sheet and roast in the oven alongside the cauliflower for 15-20 minutes, stirring halfway through.
3. In a small bowl, combine the Greek yogurt, lemon juice, and minced garlic to make the sauce. Season with salt to taste.
4. Warm the pita bread in the oven or on a skillet. Cut them in half to open the pockets.
5. Assemble the pita pockets with spinach leaves, roasted cauliflower, spiced chickpeas, and cucumber slices. Drizzle with the yogurt sauce and garnish with fresh cilantro or parsley.
6. Serve immediately.

Cold Quinoa Salad with Lemon Herb Dressing

Yield: 4 servings | **Prep time:** 15 minutes | **Cook time:** 20 minutes (for quinoa to cool)

Ingredients:

- 1 cup quinoa
- 2 cups water
- 1 cucumber, diced
- 1 bell pepper, diced
- 1/2 red onion, finely chopped
- 1 cup cherry tomatoes, halved
- 1/4 cup fresh parsley, chopped
- 1/4 cup fresh mint, chopped

For the Lemon Herb Dressing:

- 1/4 cup olive oil
- Juice of 2 lemons
- 1 garlic clove, minced
- 1 teaspoon honey or maple syrup
- Salt and pepper to taste

Nutritional Information: Estimated 300 calories, 8g protein, 45g carbohydrates, 10g fat, 5g fiber, 0mg cholesterol, 200mg sodium, 500mg potassium per serving.

Directions:

1. Rinse the quinoa under cold running water. In a medium saucepan, bring 2 cups of water to a boil. Add the quinoa, reduce heat to low, cover, and simmer for about 15 minutes or until the water is absorbed. Remove from heat and let it stand covered for 5 minutes. Fluff with a fork and allow to cool completely.
2. Combine the cooled quinoa with cucumber, bell pepper, red onion, cherry tomatoes, parsley, and mint in a large bowl.
3. Whisk together olive oil, lemon juice, minced garlic, honey (or maple syrup), salt, and pepper in a small bowl to make the dressing.
4. Pour the dressing over the quinoa salad and toss to combine thoroughly. Adjust seasoning as needed.
5. Refrigerate the salad for at least an hour before serving to allow the flavors to meld.

Vegetarian Chili with Red Lentils and Butternut Squash

Yield: 4 servings | **Prep time:** 15 minutes | **Cook time:** 35 minutes

Ingredients:

- 1 cup red lentils, rinsed
- 1 medium butternut squash, peeled, seeded, and cubed
- 1 large onion, diced
- 2 cloves garlic, minced
- 1 can (14.5 ounces) diced tomatoes
- 3 cups vegetable broth
- 1 tablespoon chili powder
- 1 teaspoon ground cumin
- 1/2 teaspoon smoked paprika
- Salt and pepper to taste
- 2 tablespoons olive oil
- Optional garnishes: chopped fresh cilantro, avocado slices, lime wedges

Nutritional Information: Estimated 320 calories, 18g protein, 55g carbohydrates, 5g fat, 15g fiber, 0mg cholesterol, 300mg sodium, 800mg potassium per serving.

Directions:

1. Heat the olive oil in a large pot over medium heat. Add the onion and garlic, sautéing until the onion is translucent, about 5 minutes.
2. Add the cubed butternut squash to the pot and cook for another 5 minutes, stirring occasionally.
3. Stir in the red lentils, diced tomatoes, vegetable broth, chili powder, cumin, smoked paprika, salt, and pepper. Bring to a boil, then reduce the heat to low and simmer, covered, for about 25 minutes or until the lentils and squash are tender.
4. Taste and adjust the seasoning as needed. If desired, serve hot, garnished with fresh cilantro, avocado slices, and lime wedges.

Smoked Turkey and Spinach Quinoa Bowl

Yield: 4 servings | **Prep time:** 10 minutes | **Cook time:** 20 minutes

Ingredients:

- 1 cup quinoa, rinsed
- 2 cups water or low-sodium vegetable broth
- 2 cups fresh spinach leaves, chopped
- 8 ounces smoked turkey breast, chopped
- 1 avocado, diced
- 1/2 cup cherry tomatoes, halved
- 1/4 cup red onion, finely diced
- 2 tablespoons olive oil
- Juice of 1 lemon
- Salt and pepper to taste
- Optional garnish: sliced almonds or pumpkin seeds

Nutritional Information: Estimated 350 calories, 22g protein, 40g carbohydrates, 14g fat, 6g fiber, 30mg cholesterol, 200mg sodium, 700mg potassium per serving.

Directions:

1. Bring the water or vegetable broth to a boil in a medium saucepan. Add the quinoa, reduce the heat to low, cover it, and simmer it for about 15 minutes until all the liquid is absorbed and the quinoa is fluffy.
2. While the quinoa is cooking, prepare the vegetables and smoked turkey. Combine the chopped spinach, diced avocado, cherry tomatoes, and red onion in a large bowl.
3. Once the quinoa is cooked, let it cool for a few minutes, then fluff it with a fork. Add the quinoa to the bowl with the vegetables and smoked turkey. Drizzle with olive oil and lemon juice, and toss to combine. Season with salt and pepper to taste.
4. Divide the quinoa mixture among serving bowls. Garnish with sliced almonds or pumpkin seeds if desired.
5. Serve immediately, or chill in the refrigerator for a cold quinoa salad.

Roasted Salmon with Farro and Brussels Sprouts

Yield: 4 servings | **Prep time:** 15 minutes | **Cook time:** 30 minutes

Ingredients:

- 4 salmon fillets (6 ounces each)
- 1 cup farro, rinsed
- 2 cups water or vegetable broth
- 3 cups Brussels sprouts, halved
- 2 tablespoons olive oil, divided
- Salt and pepper to taste
- 1 lemon, sliced into rounds
- Optional: fresh dill or parsley for garnish

Nutritional Information: Estimated 450 calories, 35g protein, 45g carbohydrates, 15g fat, 8g fiber, 75mg cholesterol, 200mg sodium, 800mg potassium per serving.

Directions:

1. Preheat the oven to 400°F (200°C). Toss the Brussels sprouts with 1 tablespoon of olive oil, salt, and pepper on a large baking sheet. Spread them out in a single layer and roast in the preheated oven for 15 minutes or until they begin to brown and soften.
2. While the Brussels sprouts are roasting, bring 2 cups of water or vegetable broth to a boil in a medium saucepan. Add the farro, reduce heat to a simmer, cover, and cook for about 25-30 minutes, or until the farro is tender and the liquid is absorbed.
3. Place the salmon fillets on the baking sheet with the Brussels sprouts after roasting for 15 minutes. Drizzle the salmon with the remaining tablespoon of olive oil and season with salt and pepper. Place lemon slices on top of the salmon.
4. Return the baking sheet to the oven and roast for 12-15 minutes, or until the salmon is cooked and flakes easily with a fork.
5. To serve, divide the cooked farro among plates and top with roasted Brussels sprouts and a salmon fillet. Garnish with fresh dill or parsley if desired.

Vegan Buddha Bowl with Tahini Dressing

Yield: 4 servings | **Prep time:** 20 minutes | **Cook time:** 30 minutes

Ingredients:

- 1 cup quinoa, rinsed
- 2 cups water
- 1 small sweet potato, cubed
- 1 cup chickpeas, drained and rinsed
- 1 avocado, sliced
- 2 cups kale, chopped
- 1 cup purple cabbage, shredded
- 1 carrot, julienned
- 2 tablespoons olive oil
- Salt and pepper to taste

For the Tahini Dressing:

- 1/4 cup tahini
- 2 tablespoons lemon juice
- 1 tablespoon maple syrup
- 2-4 tablespoons water (as needed for consistency)
- Salt to taste

Nutritional Information: Estimated 450 calories, 15g protein, 60g carbohydrates, 20g fat, 10g fiber, 0mg cholesterol, 300mg sodium, 900mg potassium per serving.

Directions:

1. Preheat the oven to 400°F (200°C). Toss the cubed sweet potato and chickpeas with olive oil, salt, and pepper. Spread them on a baking sheet and roast for 25-30 minutes, until the sweet potatoes are tender and the chickpeas are slightly crispy.
2. While the vegetables are roasting, bring 2 cups of water to a boil in a medium saucepan. Add the quinoa, reduce heat to low, cover, and simmer for about 15 minutes or until all water is absorbed. Remove from heat and let it stand covered for 5 minutes. Fluff with a fork.
3. To make the tahini dressing, whisk together tahini, lemon juice, maple syrup, and water in a small bowl until smooth. Add water as needed to achieve the desired consistency. Season with salt to taste.
4. Assemble the Buddha bowls by dividing the cooked quinoa among four bowls. Top with roasted sweet potatoes, chickpeas, avocado slices, chopped kale, shredded purple cabbage, and julienned carrot.
5. Drizzle each bowl generously with the tahini dressing before serving.

Shrimp and Mango Salad with Citrus Vinaigrette

Yield: 4 servings | **Prep time:** 20 minutes | **Cook time:** 5 minutes

Ingredients:

- 1 pound large shrimp, peeled and deveined
- 2 ripe mangoes, peeled and diced
- 1 avocado, peeled and diced
- 1/2 red onion, thinly sliced
- 1/4 cup fresh cilantro, chopped
- 8 cups mixed greens (such as arugula and spinach)

For the Citrus Vinaigrette:

- 1/4 cup olive oil
- Juice of 1 orange
- Juice of 1 lime
- 1 tablespoon honey
- Salt and pepper to taste

Nutritional Information: Estimated 350 calories, 24g protein, 30g carbohydrates, 18g fat, 5g fiber, 180mg cholesterol, 200mg sodium, 700mg potassium per serving.

Directions:

1. Heat a grill pan or skillet over medium-high heat. Cook the shrimp on each side for 2-3 minutes or until pink and opaque. Remove from heat and let cool.
2. Combine the mixed greens, diced mangoes, avocado, red onion, and cilantro in a large salad bowl. Add the cooled shrimp to the salad.
3. To make the citrus vinaigrette, whisk together the olive oil, orange juice, lime juice, honey, salt, and pepper in a small bowl until well combined.
4. Drizzle the citrus vinaigrette over the salad and toss gently to ensure all the ingredients are evenly coated.
5. Serve the salad immediately, offering additional dressing on the side if desired.

Balsamic Glazed Chicken and Roasted Vegetable Quinoa

Yield: 4 servings | **Prep time:** 15 minutes | **Cook time:** 30 minutes

Ingredients:

- 4 chicken breasts
- 1 cup quinoa
- 2 cups water
- 2 cups broccoli florets
- 1 red bell pepper, chopped
- 1 zucchini, chopped
- 1/4 cup balsamic vinegar
- 2 tablespoons olive oil, divided
- 1 tablespoon honey
- Salt and pepper to taste
- Optional: fresh thyme or basil for garnish

Nutritional Information: Estimated 450 calories, 35g protein, 45g carbohydrates, 15g fat, 6g fiber, 75mg cholesterol, 200mg sodium, 700mg potassium per serving.

Directions:

1. Preheat the oven to 425°F (220°C). Toss the broccoli, bell pepper, and zucchini with 1 tablespoon olive oil, salt, and pepper. Spread the vegetables on a baking sheet and roast for 20-25 minutes until tender and slightly caramelized.
2. While the vegetables are roasting, rinse the quinoa under cold water. In a medium saucepan, bring 2 cups of water to a boil. Add the quinoa, reduce heat to low, cover, and simmer for 15 minutes or until all water is absorbed. Remove from heat and let it sit covered for 5 minutes, then fluff with a fork.
3. Whisk together the balsamic vinegar, the remaining tablespoon of olive oil, and honey in a small bowl. Season the chicken breasts with salt and pepper. Heat a grill pan or skillet over medium-high heat, and cook the chicken for 6-7 minutes on each side or until cooked. In the last few minutes of cooking, brush the chicken with the balsamic glaze, turning to coat thoroughly.
4. Slice the glazed chicken and serve over a bed of quinoa and roasted vegetables. Drizzle any remaining balsamic glaze over the top.
5. Garnish with fresh thyme or basil if desired before serving.

Spicy Tofu Lettuce Wraps with Peanut Sauce

Yield: 4 servings | **Prep time:** 20 minutes | **Cook time:** 10 minutes

Ingredients:

- 14 ounces extra-firm tofu, drained and crumbled
- 1 tablespoon olive oil
- 1 tablespoon soy sauce
- 1 teaspoon chili flakes (adjust to taste)
- 1 garlic clove, minced
- 1 teaspoon grated ginger
- 1 head of butter lettuce, leaves separated
- 1 carrot, julienned
- 1/2 cucumber, julienned
- 1/4 cup chopped cilantro

For the Peanut Sauce:

- 1/4 cup natural peanut butter
- 2 tablespoons soy sauce
- 1 tablespoon lime juice
- 1 tablespoon honey or maple syrup
- 1 teaspoon grated ginger
- Water, as needed, to thin the sauce

Nutritional Information: Estimated 250 calories, 15g protein, 15g carbohydrates, 16g fat, 3g fiber, 0mg cholesterol, 400mg sodium, 300mg potassium per serving.

Directions:

1. Heat olive oil in a pan over medium heat. Add the crumbled tofu, soy sauce, chili flakes, garlic, and ginger. Sauté for 5-7 minutes or until the tofu is golden and slightly crispy. Remove from heat and let cool slightly.
2. While the tofu is cooking, prepare the peanut sauce by whisking together peanut butter, soy sauce, lime juice, honey (or maple syrup), and grated ginger in a bowl. Add water, one tablespoon at a time, until the sauce reaches your desired consistency.
3. Assemble the lettuce wraps by spooning the cooked tofu mixture onto a leaf. Add some julienned carrot, cucumber, and a sprinkle of chopped cilantro.
4. Drizzle each wrap with peanut sauce before serving. Serve any remaining sauce on the side for dipping.

Mediterranean Lentil and Spinach Soup

Yield: 4 servings | **Prep time:** 10 minutes | **Cook time:** 30 minutes

Ingredients:

- 1 cup dry green lentils, rinsed
- 1 tablespoon olive oil
- 1 onion, chopped
- 2 garlic cloves, minced
- 1 carrot, diced
- 1 stalk celery, diced
- 4 cups vegetable broth
- 1 can (14.5 ounces) diced tomatoes with juice
- 1 teaspoon ground cumin
- 1/2 teaspoon ground coriander
- Salt and pepper to taste
- 3 cups fresh spinach leaves
- Juice of 1 lemon
- Optional: fresh parsley or cilantro for garnish

Nutritional Information: Estimated 240 calories, 15g protein, 35g carbohydrates, 5g fat, 15g fiber, 0mg cholesterol, 300mg sodium, 700mg potassium per serving.

Directions:

1. In a large pot, heat the olive oil over medium heat. Add the onion and garlic, and sauté until the onion is translucent, about 5 minutes. Add the carrot and celery, and cook for another 5 minutes, until softened.
2. Stir in the lentils, vegetable broth, diced tomatoes with their juice, cumin, and coriander. Season with salt and pepper. Bring to a boil, then reduce the heat to low, cover, and simmer for about 20 minutes or until the lentils are tender.
3. Add the spinach to the pot and cook for another 5 minutes or until the spinach is wilted. Stir in the lemon juice.
4. Taste and adjust the seasoning as needed. Serve hot, garnished with fresh parsley or cilantro if desired.

Rainbow Vegetable and Hummus Tartine

Yield: 4 servings | **Prep time:** 15 minutes | **Cook time:** 0 minutes

Ingredients:

- 4 slices of whole grain bread (or gluten-free)
- 1 cup hummus
- 1 small beet, roasted and sliced
- 1 small carrot, peeled and shaved into ribbons
- 1/2 yellow bell pepper, thinly sliced
- 1/2 cucumber, thinly sliced
- 1/2 avocado, sliced
- 1/4 cup radishes, thinly sliced
- 1/4 cup red cabbage, shredded
- Salt and pepper to taste
- Optional: drizzle of olive oil and sprinkle of sesame seeds

Nutritional Information: Estimated 250 calories, 9g protein, 35g carbohydrates, 9g fat, 8g fiber, 0mg cholesterol, 300mg sodium, 500mg potassium per serving.

Directions:

1. Toast the whole-grain bread slices to your preferred level of crispness.
2. Spread a generous layer of hummus on each slice of toasted bread.
3. Arrange the sliced vegetables on top of the hummus in a colorful pattern, starting with beets, carrots, yellow bell peppers, cucumber, avocado, radishes, and finishing with red cabbage.
4. Season with salt and pepper to taste. Optionally, drizzle with olive oil and sprinkle sesame seeds over the top for added texture and flavor.
5. Serve immediately, enjoying the blend of creamy hummus with the crisp, fresh vegetables.

Kale Caesar Salad with Grilled Chicken

Yield: 4 servings | **Prep time:** 20 minutes | **Cook time:** 15 minutes

Ingredients:

- 4 boneless, skinless chicken breasts
- Salt and pepper to taste
- 1 tablespoon olive oil (for chicken)
- 8 cups kale, stems removed and leaves chopped
- 1/2 cup Caesar dressing, preferably made with olive oil and no added sugar
- 1/4 cup grated Parmesan cheese
- 1 cup whole-grain croutons
- Optional: lemon wedges for serving

Nutritional Information: Estimated 350 calories, 30g protein, 18g carbohydrates, 18g fat, 4g fiber, 75mg cholesterol, 500mg sodium, 600mg potassium per serving.

Directions:

1. Preheat the grill to medium-high heat. Season the chicken breasts with salt, pepper, and olive oil. Grill the chicken for 6-7 minutes on each side or until the internal temperature reaches 165°F (74°C) and the juices run clear. Let the chicken rest for a few minutes before slicing thinly.
2. Massage the kale with a bit of Caesar dressing in a large salad bowl to soften the leaves. This makes the kale more palatable and more accessible to digest.
3. Add the sliced grilled chicken to the bowl with the kale. Toss with the remaining Caesar dressing until the kale and chicken are well coated.
4. Sprinkle grated Parmesan cheese over the salad and add whole-grain croutons. Toss gently to combine.
5. Serve the salad immediately, with optional lemon wedges on the side, for a fresh, tangy finish.

Avocado, Tomato, and Cucumber Sushi Rolls

Yield: 4 servings | **Prep time:** 30 minutes | **Cook time:** 0 minutes

Ingredients:

- 2 cups sushi rice, cooked and cooled
- 4 sheets nori (seaweed)
- 1 avocado, sliced
- 1 cucumber, julienned
- 1 tomato, seeds removed and sliced into strips
- 2 tablespoons rice vinegar
- 1 tablespoon sugar
- 1/2 teaspoon salt
- Soy sauce for serving
- Pickled ginger for serving
- Wasabi, for serving

Nutritional Information: Estimated 220 calories, 6g protein, 40g carbohydrates, 5g fat, 4g fiber, 0mg cholesterol, 200mg sodium, 300mg potassium per serving.

Directions:

1. Mix the rice vinegar, sugar, and salt in a small bowl until the sugar and salt are dissolved. Gently fold this mixture into the cooked sushi rice until evenly distributed. Let the rice cool to room temperature before assembling the sushi rolls.
2. Place a sheet of nori on a bamboo sushi mat. With wet hands, spread about 1/2 cup of sushi rice evenly over the nori, leaving a small margin at the top edge of the nori sheet.
3. Arrange a few slices of avocado, cucumber, and tomato in a line on the rice, about one-third of the way up from the bottom of the nori sheet.
4. Using the bamboo mat as a guide, roll the nori tightly around the fillings, starting from the bottom and rolling up to the top edge. Moisten the top margin of the nori with water to seal the roll.
5. With a sharp knife, slice the roll into six equal pieces. Repeat the process with the remaining ingredients to make more rolls.
6. Serve the sushi rolls with soy sauce, pickled ginger, and wasabi on the side.

Tahini-Glazed Butternut Squash and Red Onion

Yield: 4 servings | **Prep time:** 15 minutes | **Cook time:** 25 minutes

Ingredients:

- 1 medium butternut squash, peeled, seeded, and cut into 1-inch cubes
- 1 large red onion, peeled and cut into wedges
- 2 tablespoons olive oil
- Salt and pepper to taste

For the Tahini Glaze:

- 1/4 cup tahini
- 2 tablespoons lemon juice
- 1 tablespoon maple syrup or honey
- 2-4 tablespoons warm water (to thin)
- Salt to taste
- Optional: sesame seeds and chopped fresh parsley for garnish

Nutritional Information: Estimated 220 calories, 4g protein, 30g carbohydrates, 11g fat, 5g fiber, 0mg cholesterol, 200mg sodium, 500mg potassium per serving.

Directions:

1. Preheat the oven to 425°F (220°C). In a large bowl, toss the butternut squash and red onion with olive oil, salt, and pepper until well coated. Spread the vegetables in a single layer on a baking sheet.
2. Roast in the preheated oven for 25 minutes, or until the butternut squash is tender and lightly caramelized, stirring halfway through the cooking time.
3. While the vegetables are roasting, prepare the tahini glaze by whisking together tahini, lemon juice, maple syrup (or honey), and warm water until smooth. Add enough water to achieve a pourable consistency. Season with salt to taste.
4. Once the vegetables are done, drizzle them with the tahini glaze and toss gently to coat.
5. Serve the vegetables garnished with sesame seeds and chopped parsley if desired.

Asian Quinoa Salad with Baked Teriyaki Salmon

Yield: 4 servings | **Prep time:** 20 minutes | **Cook time:** 20 minutes

Ingredients:

- 4 salmon fillets (6 ounces each)
- 1/4 cup teriyaki sauce (look for a low-sodium, sugar-free version)
- 1 cup quinoa
- 2 cups water
- 1 red bell pepper, diced
- 1 cup shredded carrot
- 1 cucumber, diced
- 1/4 cup sliced green onions
- 1/4 cup chopped fresh cilantro

For the Dressing:

- 2 tablespoons soy sauce (or tamari for gluten-free)
- 1 tablespoon sesame oil
- 1 tablespoon rice vinegar
- 1 teaspoon grated ginger
- 1 garlic clove, minced
- Optional: sesame seeds for garnish

Nutritional Information: Estimated 400 calories, 28g protein, 40g carbohydrates, 15g fat, 5g fiber, 60mg cholesterol, 500mg sodium, 800mg potassium per serving.

Directions:

1. Preheat the oven to 375°F (190°C). Place the salmon fillets in a baking dish and brush each fillet with teriyaki sauce. Bake for 15-20 minutes until the salmon is cooked and flakes easily with a fork.
2. While the salmon is baking, rinse the quinoa under cold running water. In a medium saucepan, bring 2 cups of water to a boil. Add the quinoa, reduce heat to low, cover, and simmer for 15 minutes or until the water is absorbed. Remove from heat and let it stand for 5 minutes, then fluff with a fork and allow it to cool slightly.
3. Combine the cooked quinoa, red bell pepper, shredded carrot, cucumber, green onions, and cilantro in a large bowl.
4. Whisk together soy sauce, sesame oil, rice vinegar, grated ginger, and minced garlic in a small bowl to make the dressing. Pour the dressing over the quinoa salad and toss to combine.
5. Divide the quinoa salad among plates and top each with a baked teriyaki salmon fillet. Garnish with sesame seeds if desired.

Spinach and Mushroom Stuffed Sweet Potatoes

Yield: 4 servings | **Prep time:** 10 minutes | **Cook time:** 45 minutes

Ingredients:

- 4 medium sweet potatoes
- 2 tablespoons olive oil, divided
- 1 garlic clove, minced
- 2 cups spinach leaves, chopped
- 1 cup mushrooms, sliced
- Salt and pepper to taste
- 1/4 cup low-sodium vegetable broth
- Optional: crumbled feta or goat cheese for topping

Nutritional Information: Estimated 220 calories, 4g protein, 40g carbohydrates, 5g fat, 6g fiber, 0mg cholesterol, 150mg sodium, 700mg potassium per serving.

Directions:

- Preheat the oven to 400°F (200°C). Prick the sweet potatoes with a fork and rub them with 1 tablespoon of olive oil. Place them on a baking sheet and bake for about 45 minutes or until tender.
- While the sweet potatoes are baking, heat the remaining tablespoon of olive oil in a large skillet over medium heat. Add the garlic and mushrooms, sautéing until the mushrooms are soft and slightly browned, about 5-7 minutes.
- Add the spinach to the skillet and cook until it wilts, about 2-3 minutes. Pour in the vegetable broth and stir until the ingredients are well combined and the liquid mostly evaporates. Season with salt and pepper to taste.
- Once the sweet potatoes are cooked, make a slit down the center of each and gently press the sides to open them up. Spoon the spinach and mushroom mixture into the sweet potatoes.
- If using, top each stuffed sweet potato with crumbled feta or goat cheese and serve immediately.

Broccoli Quinoa Casserole with Chicken

Yield: 4 servings | **Prep time:** 15 minutes | **Cook time:** 30 minutes

Ingredients:

- 1 cup quinoa, rinsed
- 2 cups low-sodium chicken broth
- 2 cups broccoli florets
- 1 pound cooked chicken breast, shredded
- 1 cup Greek yogurt
- 1 teaspoon garlic powder
- 1 teaspoon onion powder
- Salt and pepper to taste
- 1/2 cup grated Parmesan cheese
- Optional: 1/4 cup almond slivers for topping

Nutritional Information: Estimated 350 calories, 38g protein, 30g carbohydrates, 10g fat, 5g fiber, 75mg cholesterol, 300mg sodium, 500mg potassium per serving.

Directions:

1. Preheat the oven to 375°F (190°C). In a medium saucepan, bring the chicken broth to a boil. Add the quinoa, reduce the heat to low, cover, and simmer for about 15 minutes, or until the liquid is absorbed and the quinoa is fluffy.
2. Steam the broccoli florets until just tender, about 3-4 minutes, then set aside.
3. Combine the cooked quinoa, steamed broccoli, shredded chicken, Greek yogurt, garlic powder, onion powder, salt, and pepper in a large mixing bowl. Mix well until all ingredients are evenly distributed.
4. Transfer the mixture to a greased baking dish. Sprinkle the grated Parmesan cheese evenly over the top, and add almond slivers.
5. Bake in the preheated oven for about 15 minutes or until the top is golden and the casserole is heated through.
6. Serve hot, enjoying the creamy, comforting flavors of this wholesome casserole.

Mexican Quinoa Salad with Lime Cilantro Dressing

Yield: 4 servings | **Prep time**: 20 minutes | **Cook time:** 15 minutes

Ingredients:

- 1 cup quinoa, rinsed
- 2 cups water
- 1 can (15 ounces) black beans, drained and rinsed
- 1 cup corn kernels (fresh, frozen, or canned)
- 1 red bell pepper, diced
- 1 avocado, diced
- 1/2 cup cherry tomatoes, halved
- 1/4 cup red onion, finely chopped

For the Lime Cilantro Dressing:

- Juice of 2 limes
- 1/4 cup olive oil
- 1/4 cup fresh cilantro, chopped
- 1 garlic clove, minced
- 1 teaspoon honey (or maple syrup for vegan option)
- Salt and pepper to taste

Nutritional Information: Estimated 350 calories, 10g protein, 45g carbohydrates, 15g fat, 8g fiber, 0mg cholesterol, 200mg sodium, 600mg potassium per serving.

Directions:

1. In a medium saucepan, bring 2 cups of water to a boil. Add the quinoa, reduce the heat to low, cover it, and simmer it for about 15 minutes or until all the water is absorbed. Remove from heat, fluff with a fork, and let it cool to room temperature.
2. Combine the cooled quinoa, black beans, corn, red bell pepper, avocado, cherry tomatoes, and red onion in a large bowl.
3. To make the dressing, whisk together lime juice, olive oil, chopped cilantro, minced garlic, honey (or maple syrup), salt, and pepper in a small bowl until well combined.
4. Pour the dressing over the quinoa salad and toss gently to ensure everything is evenly coated.
5. Refrigerate the salad for at least 30 minutes before serving to allow the flavors to meld together.

Dinner

Turmeric Ginger Grilled Chicken

Yield: 4 servings | **Prep time:** 15 minutes (plus marinating time) | **Cook time:** 20 minutes

Ingredients:

- 4 boneless, skinless chicken breasts
- 2 tablespoons olive oil
- Juice of 1 lemon
- 1 tablespoon freshly grated ginger
- 2 teaspoons turmeric powder
- 1 garlic clove, minced
- 1 teaspoon honey
- Salt and pepper to taste
- Optional garnish: chopped fresh cilantro or parsley

Nutritional Information: Estimated 220 calories, 26g protein, 3g carbohydrates, 12g fat, 1g fiber, 75mg cholesterol, 200mg sodium, 350mg potassium per serving.

Directions:

1. Add olive oil, lemon juice, grated ginger, turmeric, minced garlic, honey, salt, and pepper to create the marinade.
2. Place the chicken breasts in a shallow dish or a resealable plastic bag. Pour the marinade over the chicken, ensuring each piece is well coated. Cover (or seal) and refrigerate for at least 2 hours or overnight for the best flavor.
3. Preheat the grill to medium-high heat. Remove the chicken from the marinade, shaking off any excess.
4. Grill the chicken for 10 minutes on each side or until the internal temperature reaches 165°F (74°C) and the juices run clear.
5. Serve the grilled chicken garnished with chopped cilantro or parsley, if desired.

Quinoa Tabbouleh with Lemon Mint Dressing

Yield: 4 servings | **Prep time:** 15 minutes | **Cook time:** 15 minutes

Ingredients:

- 1 cup quinoa, rinsed
- 2 cups water
- 1 cup cherry tomatoes, halved
- 1 cucumber, diced
- 1/2 cup red onion, finely chopped
- 1 cup fresh parsley, chopped
- 1/2 cup fresh mint, chopped

For the Lemon Mint Dressing:

- 1/4 cup olive oil
- Juice of 2 lemons
- 1 tablespoon fresh mint, finely chopped
- 1 garlic clove, minced
- Salt and pepper to taste

Nutritional Information: Estimated 280 calories, 8g protein, 38g carbohydrates, 12g fat, 6g fiber, 0mg cholesterol, 200mg sodium, 500mg potassium per serving.

Directions:

1. In a medium saucepan, bring 2 cups of water to a boil. Add the quinoa, reduce the heat to low, cover, and simmer for about 15 minutes, or until the water is absorbed and the quinoa is tender. Fluff with a fork and allow to cool to room temperature.
2. Combine the cooled quinoa, cherry tomatoes, cucumber, red onion, parsley, and mint in a large bowl.
3. To make the dressing, whisk together olive oil, lemon juice, chopped mint, minced garlic, salt, and pepper in a small bowl until well combined.
4. Pour the dressing over the quinoa mixture and toss gently to ensure everything is evenly coated.
5. Refrigerate the tabbouleh for at least 30 minutes before serving to allow the flavors to meld together.

Baked Salmon with Walnut Pesto

Yield: 4 servings | **Prep time:** 20 minutes | **Cook time:** 15 minutes

Ingredients:

- 4 salmon fillets (6 ounces each)
- Salt and pepper to taste
- 1 tablespoon olive oil

For the Walnut Pesto:

- 1/2 cup walnuts
- 2 cups fresh basil leaves
- 2 cloves garlic
- 1/2 cup grated Parmesan cheese
- 1/2 cup olive oil
- Juice of 1 lemon
- Salt and pepper to taste

Nutritional Information: Estimated 520 calories, 34g protein, 4g carbohydrates, 42g fat, 2g fiber, 75mg cholesterol, 300mg sodium, 500mg potassium per serving.

Directions:

1. Preheat the oven to 400°F (200°C). Line a baking sheet with parchment paper.
2. Season the salmon fillets with salt and pepper, and brush them with 1 tablespoon of olive oil. Place the salmon on the prepared baking sheet.
3. Bake the salmon in the preheated oven for about 12-15 minutes or until the salmon flakes easily with a fork.
4. While the salmon is baking, make the walnut pesto. Combine the walnuts, basil leaves, garlic, Parmesan cheese, lemon juice, and a pinch of salt and pepper in a food processor. Pulse until coarsely chopped. With the processor running, gradually add 1/2 cup of olive oil and continue to process until smooth.
5. Once the salmon is cooked, remove from the oven and allow to rest for a few minutes. Serve each salmon fillet with a generous spoonful of walnut pesto on top.

Sweet Potato and Black Bean Chili

Yield: 4 servings | **Prep time:** 15 minutes | **Cook time:** 30 minutes

Ingredients:

- 2 tablespoons olive oil
- 1 large onion, diced
- 2 garlic cloves, minced
- 2 medium sweet potatoes, peeled and cubed
- 1 can (15 ounces) black beans, drained and rinsed
- 1 can (14.5 ounces) diced tomatoes
- 3 cups vegetable broth
- 2 teaspoons ground cumin
- 1 teaspoon chili powder
- 1/2 teaspoon paprika
- Salt and pepper to taste
- Optional garnishes: chopped cilantro, avocado slices, lime wedges

Nutritional Information: Estimated 300 calories, 10g protein, 55g carbohydrates, 5g fat, 15g fiber, 0mg cholesterol, 200mg sodium, 800mg potassium per serving.

Directions:

1. Heat the olive oil in a large pot over medium heat. Add the onion and garlic, and sauté until the onion is translucent, about 5 minutes.
2. Add the cubed sweet potatoes to the pot and cook for another 5 minutes, stirring occasionally.
3. Stir in the black beans, diced tomatoes (with their juice), vegetable broth, cumin, chili powder, paprika, salt, and pepper. Bring the mixture to a boil, then reduce the heat to low and simmer, covered, for about 20 minutes or until the sweet potatoes are tender.
4. Taste the chili and adjust the seasoning as needed. Serve hot, garnished with chopped cilantro, avocado slices, and lime wedges if desired.

Cauliflower Steak with Tahini Sauce

Yield: 4 servings | **Prep time:** 10 minutes | **Cook time:** 25 minutes

Ingredients:

- 2 large heads of cauliflower
- 2 tablespoons olive oil
- Salt and pepper to taste

For the Tahini Sauce:

- 1/3 cup tahini
- 2 tablespoons lemon juice
- 1 garlic clove, minced
- 1/2 teaspoon sea salt
- 2-4 tablespoons water (to achieve desired consistency)
- Optional garnish: chopped parsley or sesame seeds

Nutritional Information: Estimated 220 calories, 6g protein, 15g carbohydrates, 17g fat, 5g fiber, 0mg cholesterol, 300mg sodium, 500mg potassium per serving.

Directions:

1. Preheat the oven to 425°F (220°C). Remove the leaves from the cauliflower and cut the head vertically into 1-inch thick slices, aiming to get 2-3 steaks per head, depending on size. Reserve any loose florets for another use.
2. Place the cauliflower steaks on a baking sheet. Brush both sides with olive oil and season with salt and pepper. Roast in the preheated oven for about 20-25 minutes or until tender and golden brown, flipping halfway through cooking.
3. While the cauliflower is roasting, prepare the tahini sauce. Whisk together tahini, lemon juice, minced garlic, sea salt, and water in a small bowl until smooth. Adjust the consistency with more water if needed.
4. Once the cauliflower steaks are done, place them on plates and drizzle with the tahini sauce. Garnish with chopped parsley or sesame seeds if desired.
5. Serve immediately.

Moroccan Vegetable Tagine

Yield: 4 servings | **Prep time:** 20 minutes | **Cook time:** 40 minutes

Ingredients:

- 1 tablespoon olive oil
- 1 large onion, chopped
- 2 garlic cloves, minced
- 1 teaspoon ground cumin
- 1 teaspoon ground coriander
- 1/2 teaspoon ground cinnamon
- 1/2 teaspoon turmeric
- 1/4 teaspoon cayenne pepper (adjust to taste)
- 2 cups vegetable broth
- 1 can (14.5 ounces) diced tomatoes
- 1 sweet potato, peeled and cubed
- 2 carrots, peeled and sliced
- 1 bell pepper, chopped
- 1 zucchini, sliced
- 1 cup chickpeas, drained and rinsed
- 1/2 cup dried apricots, chopped
- Salt and pepper to taste
- Optional garnish: chopped fresh cilantro or parsley

Nutritional Information: Estimated 260 calories, 8g protein, 50g carbohydrates, 4g fat, 12g fiber, 0mg cholesterol, 300mg sodium, 800mg potassium per serving.

Directions:

1. Heat the olive oil in a large pot or tagine over medium heat. Add the onion and garlic, and cook until the onion is translucent, about 5 minutes.
2. Stir in the cumin, coriander, cinnamon, turmeric, and cayenne pepper. Cook for 1-2 minutes or until fragrant.
3. Add the vegetable broth, diced tomatoes with their juice, sweet potato, carrots, and bell pepper. Bring to a boil, then reduce heat, cover, and simmer for 20 minutes.
4. Add the zucchini, chickpeas, and dried apricots to the pot. Season with salt and pepper. Cover and simmer for 15-20 minutes or until all vegetables are tender.
5. Serve the tagine hot, garnished with chopped cilantro or parsley if desired.

Mediterranean Chickpea Salad

Yield: 4 servings | **Prep time:** 15 minutes | **Cook time:** 0 minutes

Ingredients:

- 2 cans (15 ounces each) chickpeas, drained and rinsed
- 1 cucumber, diced
- 1 red bell pepper, diced
- 1/2 red onion, finely chopped
- 1 cup cherry tomatoes, halved
- 1/2 cup Kalamata olives, pitted and halved
- 1/2 cup crumbled feta cheese
- 1/4 cup fresh parsley, chopped

For the Dressing:

- 1/4 cup olive oil
- Juice of 1 lemon
- 2 garlic cloves, minced
- 1 teaspoon dried oregano
- Salt and pepper to taste

Nutritional Information: Estimated 350 calories, 12g protein, 40g carbohydrates, 18g fat, 10g fiber, 25mg cholesterol, 500mg sodium, 600mg potassium per serving.

Directions:

1. Combine chickpeas, cucumber, red bell pepper, red onion, cherry tomatoes, Kalamata olives, feta cheese, and chopped parsley in a large salad bowl.
2. To make the dressing, whisk together olive oil, lemon juice, minced garlic, dried oregano, salt, and pepper in a small bowl until well combined.
3. Pour the dressing over the salad and toss gently to ensure all ingredients are evenly coated.
4. Let the salad sit for at least 10 minutes before serving to allow the flavors to meld together.
5. Serve chilled or at room temperature.

Stuffed Bell Peppers with Quinoa and Spinach

Yield: 4 servings | **Prep time:** 20 minutes | **Cook time:** 30 minutes

Ingredients:

- 4 large bell peppers, tops cut off and seeds removed
- 1 cup quinoa, rinsed
- 2 cups vegetable broth
- 1 tablespoon olive oil
- 1 onion, diced
- 2 cloves garlic, minced
- 2 cups fresh spinach, chopped
- 1 can (15 ounces) black beans, drained and rinsed
- 1 teaspoon ground cumin
- Salt and pepper to taste
- 1/2 cup grated cheese (use a dairy-free cheese for a vegan option)
- Optional garnish: fresh cilantro, avocado slices

Nutritional Information: Estimated 320 calories, 14g protein, 50g carbohydrates, 8g fat, 10g fiber, 15mg cholesterol, 300mg sodium, 700mg potassium per serving.

Directions:

1. Preheat the oven to 375°F (190°C). Place the bell peppers in a baking dish, cut side up.
2. In a saucepan, bring the vegetable broth to a boil. Add the quinoa, reduce heat to low, cover, and simmer for about 15 minutes or until the liquid is absorbed. Remove from heat and let it sit covered for 5 minutes. Fluff the quinoa with a fork and set aside.
3. Heat the olive oil in a skillet over medium heat. Add the onion and garlic, sautéing until the onion is translucent, about 5 minutes. Add the spinach and cook until wilted, about 2-3 minutes. Stir in the cooked quinoa, black beans, cumin, salt, and pepper. Cook for an additional 2 minutes to combine the flavors.
4. Spoon the quinoa and spinach mixture into the hollowed-out bell peppers. Top with grated cheese if using.
5. Cover the baking dish with aluminum foil and bake for about 20-25 minutes until the peppers are tender. Remove the foil and bake for 5 minutes to melt the cheese.
6. Serve the stuffed peppers garnished with fresh cilantro and avocado slices if desired.

Broccoli and Almond Stir-Fry

Yield: 4 servings | **Prep time:** 10 minutes | **Cook time:** 10 minutes

Ingredients:

- 2 tablespoons olive oil
- 4 cups broccoli florets
- 1/2 cup sliced almonds
- 2 garlic cloves, minced
- 1 tablespoon ginger, minced
- 2 tablespoons soy sauce (or tamari for a gluten-free option)
- 1 tablespoon sesame oil
- 1 teaspoon honey (or maple syrup for a vegan option)
- Salt and pepper to taste
- Optional garnish: sesame seeds, green onions

Nutritional Information: Estimated 220 calories, 6g protein, 12g carbohydrates, 18g fat, 4g fiber, 0mg cholesterol, 400mg sodium, 350mg potassium per serving.

Directions:

1. Heat the olive oil in a large skillet or wok over medium-high heat. Add the broccoli florets and stir-fry for about 5 minutes or until they become tender but are still crisp.
2. Add the sliced almonds to the skillet and stir-fry for another 2-3 minutes until the almonds are golden brown.
3. Make a space in the center of the skillet, and add the minced garlic and ginger. Stir-fry for about 30 seconds or until fragrant.
4. Pour the soy sauce, sesame oil, and honey over the broccoli and almonds. Toss everything together to combine and coat the broccoli and almonds in the sauce. Season with salt and pepper to taste.
5. Cook for another 2 minutes, then remove from heat. Serve immediately, garnished with sesame seeds and chopped green onions if desired.

Grilled Eggplant with Herbed Quinoa

Yield: 4 servings | **Prep time:** 15 minutes | **Cook time:** 20 minutes

Ingredients:

- 2 medium eggplants, sliced into 1/2-inch thick rounds
- 2 tablespoons olive oil
- Salt and pepper to taste
- 1 cup quinoa, rinsed
- 2 cups vegetable broth
- 1/4 cup fresh parsley, chopped
- 1/4 cup fresh basil, chopped
- 2 tablespoons fresh lemon juice
- 1 garlic clove, minced
- 1/4 cup toasted pine nuts
- Optional garnish: crumbled feta cheese or vegan alternative

Nutritional Information: Estimated 280 calories, 8g protein, 35g carbohydrates, 14g fat, 9g fiber, 0mg cholesterol, 200mg sodium, 600mg potassium per serving.

Directions:

1. Preheat the grill to medium-high heat. Brush both sides of the eggplant slices with olive oil and season with salt and pepper. Grill the eggplant on each side for 3-4 minutes until tender and grill marks appear. Remove from the grill and set aside.
2. In a medium saucepan, bring the vegetable broth to a boil. Add the quinoa, reduce the heat to low, cover, and simmer for about 15 minutes or until the liquid is absorbed. Remove from heat, fluff with a fork, and let cool slightly.
3. Combine the cooked quinoa, parsley, basil, lemon juice, minced garlic, and pine nuts in a large bowl. Season with salt and pepper to taste, and mix well.
4. To serve, arrange the grilled eggplant slices on plates and top with the herbed quinoa mixture. If desired, garnish with crumbled feta cheese or a vegan alternative.
5. Serve warm or at room temperature.

Butternut Squash Soup with Coconut Milk

Yield: 4 servings | **Prep time:** 15 minutes | **Cook time:** 30 minutes

Ingredients:

- 1 large butternut squash (about 2 pounds), peeled, seeded, and cubed
- 2 tablespoons olive oil
- 1 medium onion, diced
- 2 garlic cloves, minced
- 1 teaspoon ground ginger
- 1/2 teaspoon ground turmeric
- 4 cups vegetable broth
- 1 can (14 ounces) coconut milk
- Salt and pepper to taste
- Optional garnish: pumpkin seeds, fresh cilantro, or a swirl of coconut milk

Nutritional Information: Estimated 250 calories, 3g protein, 30g carbohydrates, 14g fat, 6g fiber, 0mg cholesterol, 300mg sodium, 700mg potassium per serving.

Directions:

1. Heat the olive oil in a large pot over medium heat. Add the onion, garlic, and sauté until the onion is translucent and soft, about 5 minutes.
2. Add the cubed butternut squash to the pot, ground ginger, and turmeric. Cook for another 2 minutes, stirring frequently to prevent sticking, and ensure the squash is well coated with the spices.
3. Pour in the vegetable broth and bring the mixture to a boil. Reduce the heat to low, cover, and simmer for about 20 minutes or until the squash is tender and easily pierced with a fork.
4. Use an immersion blender to puree the soup until smooth. Alternatively, carefully transfer the soup to a blender and puree in batches. Return the soup to the pot if using a blender.
5. Stir in the coconut milk and season with salt and pepper to taste. Heat through on low heat, making sure not to boil the soup after adding the coconut milk.
6. Serve hot, garnished with pumpkin seeds, fresh cilantro, or a swirl of coconut milk if desired.

Spinach and Mushroom Quiche with Almond Crust

Yield: 4 servings | **Prep time:** 20 minutes | **Cook time:** 35 minutes

Ingredients:

For the Almond Crust:

- 2 cups almond flour
- 1/4 cup coconut oil, melted
- 1 egg
- 1/4 teaspoon salt

For the Filling:

- 1 tablespoon olive oil
- 1 onion, finely chopped
- 2 garlic cloves, minced
- 2 cups fresh spinach, chopped
- 1 cup mushrooms, sliced
- 4 eggs
- 1 cup almond milk
- 1/2 teaspoon salt
- 1/4 teaspoon black pepper
- 1/4 teaspoon nutmeg
- Optional: 1/2 cup grated cheese (use a dairy-free cheese for a vegan option)

Nutritional Information: Estimated 450 calories, 18g protein, 20g carbohydrates, 36g fat, 6g fiber, 210mg cholesterol, 400mg sodium, 500mg potassium per serving.

Directions:

1. Preheat the oven to 350°F (175°C). Mix almond flour, melted coconut oil, 1 egg, and 1/4 teaspoon salt in a bowl until well combined. Press the mixture into the bottom and sides of a 9-inch pie dish to form the crust. Bake for 10 minutes, then remove from the oven and set aside.
2. Heat the olive oil in a skillet over medium heat. Add the onion and garlic, and sauté until soft, about 5 minutes. Add the spinach and mushrooms, cooking until the spinach is wilted and the mushrooms are soft about 5 minutes. Spread this mixture evenly over the pre-baked crust.
3. Whisk together 4 eggs, almond milk, salt, pepper, and nutmeg in a mixing bowl. Stir in the cheese if using. Pour this egg mixture over the spinach and mushrooms into the crust.
4. Bake in the preheated oven for 25 minutes or until the filling is set and the top is slightly golden. Let the quiche cool for a few minutes before slicing.
5. Serve warm. Optional: garnish with additional fresh spinach or herbs.

Wild Salmon with Sautéed Spinach and Mushrooms

Yield: 4 servings | **Prep time:** 10 minutes | **Cook time:** 20 minutes

Ingredients:

- 4 wild salmon fillets (6 ounces each)
- 2 tablespoons olive oil, divided
- Salt and pepper to taste
- 4 cups fresh spinach leaves
- 1 cup mushrooms, sliced
- 2 garlic cloves, minced
- 1 tablespoon lemon juice
- Optional garnish: lemon slices, fresh dill

Nutritional Information: Estimated 300 calories, 34g protein, 4g carbohydrates, 17g fat, 2g fiber, 75mg cholesterol, 200mg sodium, 800mg potassium per serving.

Directions:

1. Season the salmon fillets with salt and pepper. Heat 1 tablespoon of olive oil in a large skillet over medium-high heat. Add the salmon fillets, skin-side down, and cook for about 5 minutes. Flip the fillets over and cook for another 4-5 minutes until the salmon is cooked and flakes easily with a fork. Remove from the skillet and set aside.
2. In the same skillet, add the remaining tablespoon of olive oil. Add the sliced mushrooms and sauté for about 5 minutes or until brown.
3. Add the minced garlic to the skillet and cook for another minute until fragrant. Add the spinach leaves and sauté until they wilt, about 2 minutes.
4. Stir in the lemon juice and season with additional salt and pepper to taste.
5. To serve, divide the sautéed spinach and mushrooms among plates. Top each with a salmon fillet. Garnish with lemon slices and fresh dill if desired.

Vegan Lentil Bolognese with Zoodles

Yield: 4 servings | **Prep time:** 15 minutes | **Cook time:** 30 minutes

Ingredients:

- 4 large zucchinis spiraled into noodles
- 1 cup dry red lentils, rinsed
- 2 tablespoons olive oil
- 1 onion, finely chopped
- 2 garlic cloves, minced
- 1 carrot, finely diced
- 1 celery stalk, finely diced
- 1 can (28 ounces) crushed tomatoes
- 2 teaspoons dried oregano
- 2 teaspoons dried basil
- Salt and pepper to taste
- Optional: red pepper flakes for extra heat
- Optional garnish: fresh basil leaves, nutritional yeast

Nutritional Information: Estimated 350 calories, 18g protein, 55g carbohydrates, 7g fat, 16g fiber, 0mg cholesterol, 300mg sodium, 900mg potassium per serving.

Directions:

1. Heat the olive oil in a large skillet over medium heat. Add the onion and garlic, and sauté until the onion is translucent, about 5 minutes.
2. Add the carrot and celery to the skillet, and continue to sauté for another 5 minutes or until the vegetables soften.
3. Stir in the red lentils, crushed tomatoes, oregano, basil, and red pepper flakes (if using). Season with salt and pepper. Bring the mixture to a simmer, then reduce the heat to low, cover, and cook for about 20-25 minutes, or until the lentils are tender and the sauce has thickened.
4. While the lentil bolognese is simmering, prepare the zoodles. Bring a pot of water to boil and blanch the zoodles for 1-2 minutes or until tender. Drain well.
5. Divide the zoodles among plates and top with the lentil bolognese. Garnish with fresh basil leaves and a sprinkle of nutritional yeast if desired.

Thai Coconut Curry with Tofu

Yield: 4 servings | **Prep time:** 15 minutes | **Cook time:** 20 minutes

Ingredients:

- 14 ounces of firm tofu, drained, pressed, and cut into cubes
- 2 tablespoons coconut oil
- 1 onion, sliced
- 2 garlic cloves, minced
- 1 tablespoon fresh ginger, minced
- 1 red bell pepper, sliced
- 1 carrot, julienned
- 1 zucchini, sliced
- 2 tablespoons Thai red curry paste
- 1 can (14 ounces) coconut milk
- 1 tablespoon soy sauce (or tamari for a gluten-free option)
- 1 tablespoon maple syrup
- Juice of 1 lime
- Salt to taste
- Optional garnish: fresh cilantro, sliced green onions, lime wedges
- Cooked rice or quinoa for serving

Nutritional Information: Estimated 350 calories, 12g protein, 25g carbohydrates, 24g fat, 6g fiber, 0mg cholesterol, 400mg sodium, 600mg potassium per serving.

Directions:

1. Heat the coconut oil in a large skillet or wok over medium heat. Add the tofu cubes and fry until golden on all sides, about 5-7 minutes. Remove the tofu from the skillet and set aside.
2. In the same skillet, add the onion, garlic, and ginger, and sauté until the onion is soft and translucent, about 3 minutes. Add the red bell pepper, carrot, and zucchini, cooking for another 5 minutes until the vegetables are tender.
3. Stir in the Thai red curry paste, mixing well with the vegetables for 1 minute. Pour in the coconut milk, soy sauce, and maple syrup, and bring to a gentle simmer. Let cook for 5 minutes, allowing the flavors to meld together.
4. Return the tofu to the skillet, add the lime juice, and season with salt. Stir gently to combine and heat through.
5. Serve the curry over cooked rice or quinoa, garnished with fresh cilantro, sliced green onions, and lime wedges if desired.

Roasted Brussels Sprouts with Pomegranate Glaze

Yield: 4 servings | **Prep time:** 10 minutes | **Cook time:** 25 minutes

Ingredients:

- 1.5 pounds Brussels sprouts, trimmed and halved
- 2 tablespoons olive oil
- Salt and pepper to taste
- 1/2 cup pomegranate juice
- 1 tablespoon balsamic vinegar
- 1 tablespoon honey (or maple syrup for a vegan option)
- 1/4 cup pomegranate seeds
- Optional garnish: chopped walnuts

Nutritional Information: Estimated 200 calories, 6g protein, 27g carbohydrates, 9g fat, 8g fiber, 0mg cholesterol, 200mg sodium, 500mg potassium per serving.

Directions:

1. Preheat the oven to 400°F (200°C). Toss the Brussels sprouts with olive oil, salt, and pepper on a large baking sheet until they are well coated. Spread them out in a single layer.
2. Roast in the preheated oven for about 20-25 minutes or until the Brussels sprouts are tender and crispy on the outside. Shake the pan halfway through roasting to ensure even cooking.
3. While the Brussels sprouts are roasting, combine the pomegranate juice, balsamic vinegar, and honey in a small saucepan over medium heat. Simmer until the mixture has reduced by half and has a syrup-like consistency, about 10-15 minutes.
4. Once the Brussels sprouts are roasted, transfer them to a serving dish. Drizzle the pomegranate glaze over the Brussels sprouts and toss to coat evenly.
5. Garnish with pomegranate seeds and optional chopped walnuts before serving.

Carrot Ginger Soup with Turmeric

Yield: 4 servings | **Prep time:** 10 minutes | **Cook time:** 30 minutes

Ingredients:

- 1 tablespoon coconut oil
- 1 onion, diced
- 2 tablespoons fresh ginger, minced
- 2 cloves garlic, minced
- 1 teaspoon turmeric powder
- 1.5 pounds carrots, peeled and chopped
- 4 cups vegetable broth
- Salt and pepper to taste
- Optional for garnish: coconut cream, fresh parsley or cilantro

Nutritional Information: Estimated 150 calories, 3g protein, 25g carbohydrates, 5g fat, 6g fiber, 0mg cholesterol, 500mg sodium, 700mg potassium per serving.

Directions:

1. In a large pot, heat the coconut oil over medium heat. Add the diced onion and sauté until translucent, about 5 minutes.
2. Stir in the minced ginger, garlic, and turmeric powder. Cook for another 2 minutes until fragrant.
3. Add the chopped carrots to the pot and stir until they are well-coated with the spices. Pour in the vegetable broth, and bring the mixture to a boil. Reduce heat, cover, and simmer for about 20 minutes or until the carrots are tender.
4. Puree the soup directly in the pot using an immersion blender until smooth. Alternatively, you can blend the soup in batches using a regular blender. Be careful when blending hot liquids.
5. Season the soup with salt and pepper to taste. Serve hot, garnished with a drizzle of coconut cream and a sprinkle of fresh parsley or cilantro if desired.

Baked Cod with Lemon and Dill

Yield: 4 servings | **Prep time:** 10 minutes | **Cook time:** 15 minutes

Ingredients:

- 4 cod fillets (6 ounces each)
- 2 tablespoons olive oil
- Juice and zest of 1 lemon
- 2 tablespoons fresh dill, chopped
- Salt and pepper to taste
- 4 lemon slices for garnish
- Optional: additional fresh dill for garnish

Nutritional Information: Estimated 200 calories, 23g protein, 0g carbohydrates, 10g fat, 0g fiber, 60mg cholesterol, 125mg sodium, 500mg potassium per serving.

Directions:

1. Preheat the oven to 400°F (200°C). Line a baking sheet with parchment paper or lightly grease it with olive oil.
2. Place the cod fillets on the prepared baking sheet. Brush each fillet with olive oil. Sprinkle evenly with lemon juice, zest, chopped dill, salt, and pepper.
3. Bake in the preheated oven for about 12-15 minutes, or until the fish flakes easily with a fork and is cooked through.
4. Serve immediately, garnished with lemon slices and additional fresh dill if desired.

Eggplant Parmesan with Cashew Cheese

Yield: 4 servings | **Prep time:** 20 minutes (plus soaking time for cashews) | **Cook time:** 45 minutes

Ingredients:

- 2 large eggplants, sliced into 1/2-inch thick rounds
- Salt to draw out moisture from eggplant
- 3 tablespoons olive oil
- 2 cups marinara sauce

For the Cashew Cheese:

- 1 cup raw cashews, soaked for 4 hours or overnight, then drained
- 1/4 cup water
- 2 tablespoons nutritional yeast
- 1 garlic clove
- Juice of 1/2 lemon
- Salt and pepper to taste
- Optional for layering: fresh basil leaves
- Optional for topping: vegan parmesan or additional nutritional yeast

Nutritional Information: Estimated 350 calories, 10g protein, 30g carbohydrates, 24g fat, 12g fiber, 0mg cholesterol, 600mg sodium, 800mg potassium per serving.

Directions:

1. Preheat the oven to 375°F (190°C). Sprinkle salt on both sides of the eggplant slices and let them sit for 15 minutes to draw out moisture. Pat the slices dry with paper towels to remove excess moisture and salt.
2. Brush each eggplant slice with olive oil and place on a baking sheet. Bake for 20-25 minutes, flipping halfway through, until the eggplant is tender and beginning to brown.
3. While the eggplant is baking, prepare the cashew cheese by blending soaked cashews, water, nutritional yeast, garlic, lemon juice, salt, and pepper in a blender until smooth and creamy.
4. In a baking dish, spread a thin layer of marinara sauce. Layer baked eggplant slices, a spoonful of cashew cheese, and optional fresh basil. Repeat the layers, finishing with a layer of marinara sauce. Top with vegan parmesan or additional nutritional yeast, if desired.
5. Bake in the preheated oven for 20 minutes or until the dish is heated through and the top is golden.
6. Serve hot, garnished with additional basil leaves if desired.

Ratatouille with Quinoa Pilaf

Yield: 4 servings | **Prep time:** 20 minutes | **Cook time:** 40 minutes

Ingredients:

For the Ratatouille:

- 1 eggplant, cut into 1/2-inch pieces
- 2 zucchinis, cut into 1/2-inch pieces
- 1 yellow squash, cut into 1/2-inch pieces
- 1 red bell pepper, cut into 1/2-inch pieces
- 1 yellow bell pepper, cut into 1/2-inch pieces
- 1 onion, chopped
- 3 garlic cloves, minced
- 1 can (28 ounces) diced tomatoes
- 2 tablespoons olive oil
- 1 teaspoon dried thyme
- Salt and pepper to taste

For the Quinoa Pilaf:

- 1 cup quinoa, rinsed
- 2 cups vegetable broth
- 1 tablespoon olive oil
- 1/2 onion, finely chopped
- 1 garlic clove, minced
- Salt and pepper to taste
- Optional garnish: fresh parsley or basil

Nutritional Information: Estimated 350 calories, 12g protein, 55g carbohydrates, 10g fat, 10g fiber, 0mg cholesterol, 300mg sodium, 900mg potassium per serving.

Directions:

1. For the Ratatouille: Preheat the oven to 375°F (190°C). Combine the eggplant, zucchini, yellow squash, bell peppers, onion, and garlic in a large mixing bowl. Toss with olive oil, thyme, salt, and pepper until well coated. Spread the vegetables on a baking sheet and roast for 35-40 minutes, stirring occasionally, until vegetables are tender and lightly browned.
2. For the Quinoa Pilaf: Heat 1 tablespoon of olive oil in a saucepan over medium heat while the vegetables are roasting. Add the chopped onion and minced garlic, sautéing until soft and translucent, about 5 minutes. Add the quinoa and vegetable broth, boil, then reduce heat to low, cover, and simmer for 15-20 minutes, or until the liquid is absorbed and the quinoa is tender. Fluff with a fork and season with salt and pepper to taste.
3. Combine the roasted ratatouille with the cooked quinoa pilaf, gently mixing to integrate the flavors.
4. Serve warm, garnished with fresh parsley or basil if desired.

Spaghetti Squash with Tomato Basil Sauce

Yield: 4 servings | **Prep time:** 10 minutes | **Cook time:** 40 minutes

Ingredients:

- 1 large spaghetti squash (about 2 pounds)
- 2 tablespoons olive oil, divided
- Salt and pepper to taste
- 1 onion, finely chopped
- 2 garlic cloves, minced
- 1 can (28 ounces) crushed tomatoes
- 1 teaspoon dried oregano
- 1/2 teaspoon red pepper flakes (optional)
- 1/2 cup fresh basil leaves, chopped
- Optional garnish: nutritional yeast or vegan parmesan

Nutritional Information: Estimated 220 calories, 4g protein, 30g carbohydrates, 10g fat, 6g fiber, 0mg cholesterol, 300mg sodium, 800mg potassium per serving.

Directions:

1. Preheat the oven to 400°F (200°C). Cut the spaghetti squash in half lengthwise and scoop out the seeds. Brush the inside of each half with 1 tablespoon of olive oil and season with salt and pepper. Place the squash halves cut-side down on a baking sheet and roast in the preheated oven for 30-40 minutes or until the flesh is easily pierced with a fork.
2. While the squash is roasting, heat the remaining tablespoon of olive oil in a large skillet over medium heat. Add the onion and garlic, and sauté until the onion is translucent, about 5 minutes.
3. Add the crushed tomatoes, oregano, and red pepper flakes to the skillet. Simmer the sauce for 20 minutes, stirring occasionally. Season with salt and pepper to taste.
4. Once the spaghetti squash is cooked and cool enough to handle, use a fork to scrape the inside flesh into strands, creating the "spaghetti".
5. Serve the spaghetti squash topped with the tomato basil sauce. Garnish with chopped fresh basil and optional nutritional yeast or vegan parmesan.

Rainbow Vegetable Stir-Fry with Tamari Sauce

Yield: 4 servings | **Prep time:** 15 minutes | **Cook time:** 10 minutes

Ingredients:

- 1 tablespoon sesame oil
- 1 red bell pepper, sliced
- 1 yellow bell pepper, sliced
- 1 orange bell pepper, sliced
- 1 cup broccoli florets
- 1 cup snap peas
- 1 carrot, julienned
- 1 small purple cabbage, shredded
- 2 green onions, sliced
- 1 tablespoon fresh ginger, minced
- 2 garlic cloves, minced
- 1/4 cup tamari sauce (gluten-free soy sauce)
- 1 tablespoon maple syrup
- 1 teaspoon rice vinegar
- Optional for serving: sesame seeds, cooked quinoa or brown rice

Nutritional Information: Estimated 150 calories, 4g protein, 20g carbohydrates, 5g fat, 4g fiber, 0mg cholesterol, 600mg sodium, 400mg potassium per serving.

Directions:

1. Heat the sesame oil in a large skillet or wok over medium-high heat. Add the red, yellow, and orange bell peppers, broccoli, snap peas, carrots, and purple cabbage. Stir-fry for 5-7 minutes or until the vegetables are tender but crisp.
2. Make a well in the center of the skillet, and add the green onions, ginger, and garlic. Stir-fry for an additional minute until fragrant.
3. Whisk together the tamari sauce, maple syrup, and rice vinegar in a small bowl. Pour this sauce over the vegetables and toss to combine, ensuring all the vegetables are coated evenly with the sauce.
4. Cook for another 2 minutes, then remove from heat. Serve hot cooked quinoa or brown rice, garnished with sesame seeds if desired.

Roasted Garlic Cauliflower Mash

Yield: 4 servings | **Prep time:** 10 minutes | **Cook time:** 40 minutes

Ingredients:

- 1 large head of cauliflower, cut into florets
- 1 whole garlic bulb
- 2 tablespoons olive oil, divided
- Salt and pepper to taste
- 1/4 cup almond milk (or any plant-based milk)
- 2 tablespoons nutritional yeast (optional for a cheesy flavor)
- 1 teaspoon fresh thyme leaves (optional)

Nutritional Information: Estimated 120 calories, 4g protein, 12g carbohydrates, 7g fat, 5g fiber, 0mg cholesterol, 150mg sodium, 500mg potassium per serving.

Directions:

1. Preheat the oven to 400°F (200°C). Toss the cauliflower florets with 1 tablespoon of olive oil, salt, and pepper. Spread the florets in a single layer on a baking sheet. Cut the top off the garlic bulb to expose the cloves, drizzle with the remaining olive oil, wrap in foil, and place on the baking sheet with the cauliflower.
2. Roast in the preheated oven for about 30-35 minutes, or until the cauliflower is tender and slightly golden and the garlic is soft.
3. Once roasted, squeeze the garlic cloves out of their skins into a food processor. Add the roasted cauliflower, almond milk, and nutritional yeast (if using), and blend until smooth and creamy. You may need to scrape down the sides a few times. Adjust the almond milk to achieve your desired consistency.
4. Taste and adjust the seasoning with additional salt and pepper if needed. Stir in fresh thyme leaves if using.
5. Serve the cauliflower mash hot as a side dish.

Cilantro Lime Chicken with Avocado Salsa

Yield: 4 servings | **Prep time:** 20 minutes | **Cook time:** 15 minutes

Ingredients:

- 4 boneless, skinless chicken breasts
- 2 tablespoons olive oil
- Juice and zest of 2 limes
- 1/4 cup fresh cilantro, chopped
- 2 garlic cloves, minced
- 1/2 teaspoon chili powder
- Salt and pepper to taste

For the Avocado Salsa:

- 2 ripe avocados, diced
- 1 small red onion, finely chopped
- 1 tomato, diced
- Juice of 1 lime
- 1/4 cup fresh cilantro, chopped
- Salt and pepper to taste

Nutritional Information: Estimated 350 calories, 26g protein, 14g carbohydrates, 22g fat, 7g fiber, 75mg cholesterol, 200mg sodium, 800mg potassium per serving.

Directions:

1. Whisk together olive oil, lime juice, zest, chopped cilantro, minced garlic, chili powder, salt, and pepper in a bowl. Place the chicken breasts in the marinade and ensure they are well coated. Let marinate in the refrigerator for at least 30 minutes or up to 4 hours for more flavor.
2. Preheat a grill or grill pan over medium-high heat. Remove the chicken from the marinade, shaking off any excess. Grill the chicken for 6-7 minutes on each side or until fully cooked and the internal temperature reaches 165°F (74°C).
3. While the chicken is cooking, prepare the avocado salsa. Combine diced avocados, chopped red onion, tomato, lime juice, chopped cilantro, salt, and pepper in a medium bowl. Gently toss to combine without mashing the avocados.
4. Once the chicken is cooked, let it rest for a few minutes before slicing. Serve the chicken topped with the avocado salsa.
5. Optional: Serve with additional lime wedges and a sprinkle of fresh cilantro.

Grilled Shrimp Salad with Citrus Dressing

Yield: 4 servings | **Prep time:** 15 minutes | **Cook time:** 10 minutes

Ingredients:

- 1 pound large shrimp, peeled and deveined
- 1 tablespoon olive oil
- Salt and pepper to taste
- 8 cups mixed greens (such as spinach, arugula, and romaine)
- 1 avocado, sliced
- 1 orange, segmented
- 1/2 red onion, thinly sliced

For the Citrus Dressing:

- Juice of 1 orange
- Juice of 1 lemon
- 2 tablespoons olive oil
- 1 tablespoon honey (or maple syrup for vegan option)
- 1 teaspoon Dijon mustard
- Salt and pepper to taste

Nutritional Information: Estimated 320 calories, 24g protein, 18g carbohydrates, 18g fat, 6g fiber, 180mg cholesterol, 300mg sodium, 700mg potassium per serving.

Directions:

1. Preheat the grill or a grill pan to medium-high heat. Toss the shrimp with 1 tablespoon olive oil, salt, and pepper. Grill the shrimp on each side for 2-3 minutes or until they are pink and opaque. Remove from the grill and set aside to cool slightly.
2. Combine the mixed greens, sliced avocado, orange segments, and thinly sliced red onion in a large salad bowl.
3. To make the citrus dressing, whisk together orange juice, lemon juice, olive oil, honey (or maple syrup), Dijon mustard, salt, and pepper in a small bowl until well combined.
4. Drizzle the citrus dressing over the salad and toss it to coat it evenly. Top the salad with the grilled shrimp.
5. Serve immediately, offering additional dressing on the side if desired.

Pineapple Teriyaki Chicken Skewers

Yield: 4 servings | **Prep time:** 30 minutes (including marination) | **Cook time:** 15 minutes

Ingredients:

- 1 pound chicken breast, cut into 1-inch cubes
- 1 cup fresh pineapple, cut into 1-inch cubes
- 1 large bell pepper (any color), cut into 1-inch pieces
- 1 large red onion, cut into 1-inch pieces

For the Teriyaki Sauce:

- 1/4 cup tamari (gluten-free soy sauce)
- 1/4 cup water
- 2 tablespoons honey (or maple syrup for a vegan option)
- 1 garlic clove, minced
- 1 teaspoon fresh ginger, grated
- 1 tablespoon cornstarch mixed with 2 tablespoons water (for thickening)
- Wooden or metal skewers

Nutritional Information: Estimated 250 calories, 26g protein, 20g carbohydrates, 6g fat, 2g fiber, 65mg cholesterol, 700mg sodium, 400mg potassium per serving.

Directions:

1. Combine tamari, water, honey (or maple syrup), garlic, and ginger in a small saucepan. Bring to a simmer over medium heat. Stir in the cornstarch mixture and continue to simmer until the sauce thickens about 2-3 minutes. Remove from heat and let cool.
2. Reserve half of the teriyaki sauce for serving. In the refrigerator, use the other half to marinate the chicken cubes for at least 20 minutes.
3. Preheat the grill to medium-high heat. If using wooden skewers, soak them in water for at least 30 minutes to prevent burning.
4. Thread the marinated chicken, pineapple, bell pepper, and red onion onto the skewers, alternating between them.
5. Grill the skewers on each side for 5-7 minutes, or until the chicken is cooked and the vegetables are slightly charred, brushing occasionally with the teriyaki sauce.
6. Serve the skewers with the reserved teriyaki sauce for dipping.

Lemon Herb Roasted Chicken with Asparagus

Yield: 4 servings | **Prep time:** 15 minutes | **Cook time:** 45 minutes

Ingredients:

- 4 chicken breasts, bone-in, and skin-on
- 1 pound asparagus, ends trimmed
- 2 lemons, one sliced and one juiced
- 2 tablespoons olive oil
- 4 garlic cloves, minced
- 1 tablespoon fresh rosemary, chopped
- 1 tablespoon fresh thyme, chopped
- Salt and pepper to taste

Nutritional Information: Estimated 300 calories, 35g protein, 10g carbohydrates, 14g fat, 3g fiber, 95mg cholesterol, 200mg sodium, 500mg potassium per serving.

Directions:

1. Preheat the oven to 375°F (190°C). Arrange the chicken breasts in a large baking dish. Scatter the asparagus around the chicken.
2. Whisk together olive oil, lemon juice, minced garlic, rosemary, thyme, salt, and pepper in a small bowl. Pour this mixture evenly over the chicken and asparagus, ensuring each piece is well-coated.
3. Place lemon slices over the chicken and around the dish.
4. Roast in the preheated oven for about 35-45 minutes, or until the chicken is cooked through (reaching an internal temperature of 165°F or 74°C) and the asparagus is tender.
5. Halfway through the cooking time, baste the chicken and asparagus with the juices collected at the bottom of the dish.
6. Serve hot, garnished with additional fresh herbs if desired.

Artichoke and Spinach Stuffed Portobellos

Yield: 4 servings | **Prep time:** 15 minutes | **Cook time:** 20 minutes

Ingredients:

- 4 large portobello mushroom caps, stems, and gills removed
- 2 tablespoons olive oil, divided
- Salt and pepper to taste
- 1 small onion, finely chopped
- 2 garlic cloves, minced
- 1 can (14 ounces) artichoke hearts, drained and chopped
- 2 cups fresh spinach, roughly chopped
- 1/2 cup cashew nuts, soaked for 2 hours and drained
- 1/4 cup nutritional yeast
- 1 tablespoon lemon juice
- 1/2 teaspoon dried oregano
- Optional garnish: fresh parsley, chopped

Nutritional Information: Estimated 250 calories, 8g protein, 18g carbohydrates, 18g fat, 5g fiber, 0mg cholesterol, 300mg sodium, 600mg potassium per serving.

Directions:

1. Preheat the oven to 375°F (190°C). Brush the portobello mushroom caps with 1 tablespoon of olive oil and season with salt and pepper. Place them gill-side on a baking sheet and roast for 10 minutes until slightly softened.
2. While the mushrooms are roasting, heat the remaining tablespoon of olive oil in a skillet over medium heat. Add the onion and garlic, sautéing until soft and translucent, about 5 minutes. Add the chopped artichoke hearts and spinach, cooking until the spinach is wilted, about 3 minutes. Remove from heat.
3. Combine the soaked cashew nuts, nutritional yeast, lemon juice, oregano, and a pinch of salt and pepper in a blender. Blend until smooth, adding a little water to achieve a creamy consistency.
4. Remove the mushrooms from the oven and flip them over. Fill each mushroom cap with the spinach-artichoke mixture, then top with a layer of the cashew cream.
5. Return the stuffed mushrooms to the oven and bake for 10 minutes until the filling is heated and the tops are golden.
6. Serve hot, garnished with chopped fresh parsley if desired.

Vegan Paella with Saffron and Seasonal Vegetables

Yield: 4 servings | **Prep time:** 15 minutes | **Cook time:** 35 minutes

Ingredients:

- 1 tablespoon olive oil
- 1 large onion, diced
- 2 garlic cloves, minced
- 1 red bell pepper, sliced
- 1 yellow bell pepper, sliced
- 1 cup green beans, trimmed and cut into 1-inch pieces
- 1 cup artichoke hearts, quartered (fresh or canned)
- 1/2 cup frozen peas, thawed
- 2 cups short-grain rice, such as Arborio or Bomba
- 4 cups vegetable broth
- 1/4 teaspoon saffron threads, crushed
- 1 teaspoon smoked paprika
- 1 teaspoon turmeric
- Salt and pepper to taste
- Lemon wedges for serving
- Fresh parsley, chopped, for garnish

Nutritional Information: Estimated 350 calories, 9g protein, 65g carbohydrates, 5g fat, 7g fiber, 0mg cholesterol, 700mg sodium, 400mg potassium per serving.

Directions:

- Heat the olive oil in a large skillet or paella pan over medium heat. Add the onion and garlic, sautéing until the onion is translucent, about 5 minutes.
- Add the red and yellow bell peppers, green beans, and artichoke hearts to the pan. Cook for another 5 minutes, stirring occasionally, until the vegetables soften.
- Stir in the rice, ensuring it is well coated with the oil and mixed with the vegetables. Cook for 2 minutes.
- Pour in the vegetable broth, then add the saffron, smoked paprika, turmeric, salt, and pepper. Stir well to distribute the spices and saffron. Bring to a simmer, then reduce the heat to low. Cover and cook for about 20-25 minutes until the rice is tender and the liquid has been absorbed.
- Sprinkle the thawed peas over the rice five minutes before the end of cooking. Do not stir; just let them heat through.
- Once cooked, remove the paella from the heat and let it sit covered for 5 minutes. Serve with lemon wedges and garnish with fresh parsley.

Grilled Asparagus and Fennel Salad

Yield: 4 servings | **Prep time:** 15 minutes | **Cook time:** 10 minutes

Ingredients:

- 1 pound asparagus, trimmed
- 1 large fennel bulb, thinly sliced
- 2 tablespoons olive oil
- Salt and pepper to taste
- 2 tablespoons lemon juice
- 1 teaspoon Dijon mustard
- 1 garlic clove, minced
- 1/4 cup shaved Parmesan cheese (optional for vegan, use nutritional yeast)
- 1/4 cup toasted pine nuts
- Fresh parsley, chopped, for garnish

Nutritional Information: Estimated 180 calories, 6g protein, 10g carbohydrates, 14g fat, 5g fiber, 5mg cholesterol, 200mg sodium, 400mg potassium per serving.

Directions:

1. Preheat the grill to medium-high heat. Toss the asparagus and fennel slices with 1 tablespoon of olive oil, salt, and pepper in a bowl until they are evenly coated.
2. Grill the asparagus and fennel for about 5-7 minutes, turning occasionally, until they are charred antender but still crisp.
3. Whisk together the remaining olive oil, lemon juice, Dijon mustard, minced garlic, salt, and pepper in a small bowl to create the dressing.
4. Arrange the grilled asparagus and fennel on a serving platter. Drizzle with the lemon mustard dressing.
5. Top the salad with shaved Parmesan cheese (or nutritional yeast), toasted pine nuts, and fresh parsley before serving.

Lemon Pepper Trout with Garlic Spinach

Yield: 4 servings | **Prep time:** 10 minutes | **Cook time:** 20 minutes

Ingredients:

- 4 trout fillets (about 6 ounces each)
- 2 tablespoons olive oil, divided
- 1 tablespoon lemon pepper seasoning
- Salt to taste
- 4 cups fresh spinach leaves
- 4 garlic cloves, minced
- Juice of 1 lemon
- Optional garnish: lemon slices and fresh parsley

Nutritional Information: Estimated 250 calories, 28g protein, 3g carbohydrates, 14g fat, 1g fiber, 75mg cholesterol, 200mg sodium, 500mg potassium per serving.

Directions:

1. Preheat your oven to 400°F (200°C). Line a baking sheet with parchment paper.
2. Place the trout fillets on the prepared baking sheet. Brush each fillet with 1 tablespoon of olive oil, then sprinkle evenly with lemon pepper seasoning and a pinch of salt.
3. Bake the trout in the preheated oven for about 12-15 minutes or until the fish flakes easily with a fork.
4. While the trout is baking, heat the remaining tablespoon of olive oil in a large skillet over medium heat. Add the minced garlic and sauté for 1 minute until fragrant but not browned.
5. Add the spinach to the skillet, tossing it with the garlic and oil. Cook for 2-3 minutes or until the spinach is wilted. Season with salt to taste and squeeze fresh lemon juice over the cooked spinach.
6. Serve the baked trout fillets with the garlic spinach on the side. Garnish with lemon slices and fresh parsley if desired.

Desserts

Avocado Chocolate Mousse

Yield: 4 servings | **Prep time:** 15 minutes | **Cook time:** 0 minutes

Ingredients:

- 2 ripe avocados, peeled and pitted
- 1/4 cup unsweetened cocoa powder
- 1/4 cup maple syrup or honey (adjust to taste)
- 1/2 teaspoon vanilla extract
- A pinch of salt
- 1/4 cup almond milk (or any plant-based milk), adjust as needed for consistency
- Optional for garnish: fresh berries, shaved dark chocolate, or chopped nuts

Nutritional Information: Estimated 250 calories, 4g protein, 30g carbohydrates, 15g fat, 10g fiber, 0mg cholesterol, 100mg sodium, 500mg potassium per serving.

Directions:

1. In a food processor or high-speed blender, combine the avocados, cocoa powder, maple syrup (or honey), vanilla extract, and a pinch of salt. Blend until the mixture is smooth and creamy.
2. While blending, gradually add the almond milk until you reach your desired consistency. The mousse should be thick and creamy.
3. Taste the mousse and adjust the sweetness if necessary by adding a little more maple syrup or honey.
4. Divide the mousse into serving dishes and refrigerate for at least 1 hour to chill and set.
5. If desired, serve chilled, garnished with fresh berries, shaved dark chocolate, or chopped nuts.

Coconut Chia Seed Pudding

Yield: 4 servings | **Prep time:** 10 minutes (plus 4 hours for chilling) | **Cook time:** 0 minutes

Ingredients:

- 1/3 cup chia seeds
- 1 can (14 ounces) full-fat coconut milk
- 2 tablespoons maple syrup or honey
- 1/2 teaspoon vanilla extract
- A pinch of salt
- Optional for serving: Fresh berries, sliced banana, toasted coconut flakes, or nuts

Nutritional Information: Estimated 280 calories, 5g protein, 18g carbohydrates, 22g fat, 8g fiber, 0mg cholesterol, 50mg sodium, 300mg potassium per serving.

Directions:

1. In a mixing bowl, whisk together the coconut milk, maple syrup (or honey), vanilla extract, and a pinch of salt until well combined.
2. Stir in the chia seeds until evenly distributed. Let the mixture sit for 5 minutes, then stir again to prevent the chia seeds from clumping.
3. Cover the bowl with plastic wrap or transfer the mixture into a sealable container. Refrigerate for at least 4 hours, or overnight, until the chia seeds have absorbed the liquid and the pudding has thickened.
4. Before serving, stir the pudding to check the consistency. If it's too thick, you can thin it with a little more coconut milk or water.
5. Serve the chia pudding in individual bowls or glasses, topped with your choice of fresh berries, sliced banana, toasted coconut flakes, or nuts.

Spiced Baked Apples with Walnuts

Yield: 4 servings | **Prep time:** 15 minutes | **Cook time:** 30 minutes

Ingredients:

- 4 large apples, such as Fuji or Honeycrisp
- 1/4 cup walnuts, chopped
- 2 tablespoons maple syrup
- 1/2 teaspoon ground cinnamon
- 1/4 teaspoon ground nutmeg
- 1/4 teaspoon ground ginger
- 1/4 cup water
- Optional: A pinch of ground cloves

Nutritional Information: Estimated 200 calories, 2g protein, 34g carbohydrates, 7g fat, 5g fiber, 0mg cholesterol, 5mg sodium, 250mg potassium per serving.

Directions:

1. Preheat the oven to 350°F (175°C). Core the apples, leaving the bottom intact to create a well for the filling.
2. In a small bowl, mix the chopped walnuts, maple syrup, cinnamon, nutmeg, ginger, and cloves (if using) until well combined.
3. Stuff each apple with the walnut-spice mixture, dividing it evenly among the apples.
4. Place the stuffed apples in a baking dish. Pour water into the bottom of the dish to help steam the apples as they bake.
5. Bake in the preheated oven for about 30 minutes or until the apples are tender but not mushy. Baste the apples occasionally with the liquid from the bottom of the dish.
6. Serve warm, with the syrupy juices spooned over the top of each apple.

Almond Flour Lemon Bars

Yield: 6 servings | **Prep time:** 15 minutes | **Cook time:** 25 minutes

Ingredients:

For the crust:

- 2 cups almond flour
- 1/3 cup coconut oil, melted
- 2 tablespoons maple syrup
- A pinch of salt

For the lemon filling:

- 3 large eggs
- 1/2 cup lemon juice (about 2-3 lemons)
- Zest of 1 lemon
- 1/2 cup maple syrup
- 2 tablespoons almond flour

Nutritional Information: Estimated 350 calories, 10g protein, 30g carbohydrates, 24g fat, 4g fiber, 93mg cholesterol, 45mg sodium, 200mg potassium per serving.

Directions:

1. Preheat the oven to 350°F (175°C). Line an 8x8-inch baking dish with parchment paper, leaving some overhang for easy removal.
2. Make the crust: In a mixing bowl, combine 2 cups almond flour, melted coconut oil, 2 tablespoons maple syrup, and a pinch of salt. Mix until a dough forms. Press the dough evenly into the bottom of the prepared baking dish. Bake for 10-12 minutes, or until lightly golden. Remove from the oven and let cool slightly.
3. Make the lemon filling: In a separate bowl, whisk together the eggs, lemon juice, lemon zest, 1/2 cup maple syrup, and 2 tablespoons almond flour until smooth. Pour the filling over the baked crust.
4. Return to the oven and bake for 12-15 minutes or until the filling is set but still slightly jiggly in the center.
5. Remove from the oven and let cool completely at room temperature. Then, chill in the refrigerator for at least 2 hours before slicing into bars.
6. Serve chilled, optionally dusted with powdered erythritol or garnished with lemon zest.

No-Bake Cashew Vanilla Bean Cheesecake

Yield: 6 servings | **Prep time:** 20 minutes (plus soaking time & chilling time) | **Cook time:** 0 minutes

Ingredients:

For the crust:

- 1 cup raw almonds
- 1 cup pitted dates, soaked in warm water for 10 minutes and drained
- A pinch of sea salt

For the filling:

- 2 cups raw cashews, soaked in water for 4 hours or overnight, then drained
- 1/2 cup coconut cream
- 1/4 cup maple syrup
- Juice of 1 lemon
- 1 vanilla bean, split and scraped, or 1 teaspoon pure vanilla extract
- A pinch of sea salt

Nutritional Information: Estimated 450 calories, 12g protein, 40g carbohydrates, 30g fat, 5g fiber, 0mg cholesterol, 100mg sodium, 600mg potassium per serving.

Directions:

1. Prepare the crust: In a food processor, pulse almonds, soaked dates, and a pinch of sea salt until the mixture sticks together when pressed between fingers. Press the mixture firmly into the bottom of a lined 6-inch springform pan or a pie dish and set aside.
2. Make the filling: In a high-speed blender, combine soaked and drained cashews, coconut cream, maple syrup, lemon juice, vanilla bean seeds (or vanilla extract), and a pinch of sea salt. Blend on high until the mixture is completely smooth and creamy, scraping down the sides as necessary.
3. Pour the filling over the crust and smooth the top with a spatula. Cover and freeze for at least 4 hours or until firm.
4. Before serving, remove the cheesecake from the freezer and let it sit at room temperature for about 10 minutes to soften slightly. Slice and serve chilled.
5. Optional: Garnish with fresh berries, lemon zest, or a drizzle of honey before serving.

Blueberry Oat Crumble Bars

Yield: 6 servings | **Prep time:** 15 minutes | **Cook time:** 25 minutes

Ingredients:

For the crust and crumble:

- 2 cups rolled oats (or gluten-free oatmeal)
- 1 cup almond flour
- 1/4 cup coconut oil, melted
- 1/4 cup maple syrup
- 1 teaspoon vanilla extract
- A pinch of salt

For the filling:

- 2 cups fresh blueberries
- 2 tablespoons chia seeds
- 2 tablespoons maple syrup
- 1 teaspoon lemon zest
- Juice of 1/2 lemon

Nutritional Information: Estimated 300 calories, 6g protein, 35g carbohydrates, 15g fat, 6g fiber, 0mg cholesterol, 30mg sodium, 200mg potassium per serving.

Directions:

1. Preheat the oven to 350°F (175°C). Line an 8x8-inch baking dish with parchment paper.
2. In a large bowl, mix the rolled oats, almond flour, melted coconut oil, maple syrup, vanilla extract, and a pinch of salt until well combined. Reserve 1/2 cup of this mixture for the topping.
3. Press the remaining mixture firmly into the bottom of the prepared baking dish to form the crust.
4. Combine the blueberries, chia seeds, maple syrup, lemon zest, and lemon juice in another bowl. Spread this mixture evenly over the crust.
5. Sprinkle the reserved 1/2 cup of the oat mixture over the blueberry layer.
6. Bake in the preheated oven for 25 minutes or until the top is lightly golden and the filling is bubbly.
7. Let the bars cool completely in the dish before cutting into squares.

Vegan Mango Sorbet

Yield: 4 servings | **Prep time:** 10 minutes (plus freezing time) | **Cook time:** 0 minutes

Ingredients:

- 3 large ripe mangoes, peeled and cubed
- 1/4 cup fresh lime juice
- 1/3 cup maple syrup or to taste
- 1/2 cup water

Nutritional Information: Estimated 150 calories, 1g protein, 38g carbohydrates, 0g fat, 3g fiber, 0mg cholesterol, 1mg sodium, 300mg potassium per serving.

Directions:

1. Place the cubed mangoes in a freezer-safe container and freeze until solid, about 4 hours or overnight.
2. Once the mangoes are frozen, place them in a food processor or high-powered blender. Add the lime juice, maple syrup, and water.
3. Blend on high until the mixture is smooth and creamy. You may need to stop and scrape down the sides a few times to ensure everything is well combined. If the sorbet is too thick, you can add a little more water to reach the desired consistency.
4. Taste the sorbet and adjust the sweetness if necessary by adding a bit more maple syrup. Blend again if an additional sweetener is added.
5. Serve immediately for a soft-serve texture, or transfer the sorbet to a freezer-safe container and freeze for another 1-2 hours for a firmer consistency.
6. Scoop into bowls or cones and enjoy!

Baked Peaches with Cinnamon and Nutmeg

Yield: 4 servings | **Prep time:** 10 minutes | **Cook time:** 25 minutes

Ingredients:

- 4 ripe peaches, halved and pitted
- 2 tablespoons coconut oil, melted
- 2 tablespoons maple syrup
- 1/2 teaspoon ground cinnamon
- 1/4 teaspoon ground nutmeg
- Optional for serving: A dollop of coconut yogurt or a sprinkle of chopped nuts

Nutritional Information: Estimated 150 calories, 1g protein, 20g carbohydrates, 7g fat, 3g fiber, 0mg cholesterol, 0mg sodium, 300mg potassium per serving.

Directions:

1. Preheat the oven to 375°F (190°C). Arrange the peach halves cut side up in a baking dish.
2. Combine the melted coconut oil, maple syrup, cinnamon, and nutmeg in a small bowl. Mix well.
3. Spoon the mixture over each peach half, evenly distributing the spices.
4. Bake in the preheated oven for about 25 minutes or until the peaches are tender and the tops are slightly caramelized.
5. Serve warm, optionally topped with a dollop of coconut yogurt or a sprinkle of chopped nuts for added texture and flavor.

Raspberry Coconut Macaroons

Yield: 4 servings | **Prep time:** 15 minutes | **Cook time:** 20 minutes

Ingredients:

- 1 1/2 cups unsweetened shredded coconut
- 1/2 cup fresh raspberries
- 1/4 cup maple syrup
- 2 tablespoons coconut flour
- 1 teaspoon vanilla extract
- A pinch of salt
- 2 egg whites

Nutritional Information: Estimated 200 calories, 3g protein, 18g carbohydrates, 14g fat, 5g fiber, 0mg cholesterol, 60mg sodium, 200mg potassium per serving.

Directions:

1. Preheat the oven to 325°F (163°C) and line a baking sheet with parchment paper.
2. In a food processor, pulse the raspberries until they are broken into a puree.
3. In a large bowl, mix the shredded coconut, raspberry puree, maple syrup, coconut flour, vanilla extract, and a pinch of salt until well combined.
4. In a separate bowl, beat the egg whites until stiff peaks form. Gently fold the egg whites into the coconut mixture.
5. Use a tablespoon or a cookie scoop to form the mixture into small mounds on the prepared baking sheet, spacing them about an inch apart.
6. Bake in the preheated oven for 18-20 minutes or until the edges are golden brown.
7. Let the macaroons cool on the baking sheet for 10 minutes, then transfer to a wire rack to cool completely.

Matcha Green Tea Coconut Ice Cream

Yield: 4 servings | **Prep time:** 15 minutes (plus chilling and freezing time) | **Cook time:** 0 minutes

Ingredients:

- 1 can (14 ounces) full-fat coconut milk, chilled overnight
- 1/4 cup maple syrup or honey
- 2 teaspoons matcha green tea powder
- 1 teaspoon vanilla extract
- A pinch of salt

Nutritional Information: Estimated 300 calories, 3g protein, 20g carbohydrates, 25g fat, 0g fiber, 0mg cholesterol, 15mg sodium, 200mg potassium per serving.

Directions:

1. Open the chilled can of coconut milk and scoop the solidified cream into a mixing bowl, leaving any liquid behind (this can be used in smoothies).
2. Add the maple syrup (or honey), matcha green tea powder, vanilla extract, and a pinch of salt to the bowl.
3. Use an electric mixer to beat the mixture on high speed until it is smooth and well combined. Taste and adjust sweetness if necessary.
4. Transfer the mixture to a loaf pan or a freezer-safe container. Cover and freeze for at least 4 hours or until firm.
5. Before serving, let the ice cream sit at room temperature for a few minutes to soften slightly for easier scooping.
6. Serve in bowls or cones, garnished with a sprinkle of matcha powder or shaved chocolate if desired.

Pumpkin Spice Chia Pudding

Yield: 4 servings | **Prep time:** 15 minutes | **Cook time:** 0 minutes (plus at least 4 hours for chilling)

Ingredients:

- 1/4 cup chia seeds
- 1 cup unsweetened almond milk
- 3/4 cup pumpkin puree (not pumpkin pie filling)
- 2 tablespoons maple syrup, or to taste
- 1 teaspoon vanilla extract
- 3/4 teaspoon pumpkin pie spice
- A pinch of salt

Nutritional Information: Estimated 150 calories, 4g protein, 25g carbohydrates, 4g fat, 7g fiber, 0mg cholesterol, 55mg sodium, 350mg potassium per serving.

Directions:

1. In a medium bowl, whisk the almond milk, pumpkin puree, maple syrup, vanilla extract, pumpkin pie spice, and a pinch of salt until well combined.
2. Add the chia seeds to the pumpkin mixture, stirring thoroughly to ensure the seeds are evenly distributed.
3. Cover the bowl with a lid or plastic wrap and refrigerate for at least 4 hours, or overnight, until the pudding has thickened and the chia seeds have absorbed the liquid.
4. Before serving, stir the pudding to break up any clumps. If the pudding is too thick, you can adjust its consistency by adding a little more almond milk.
5. Serve the chia pudding in individual bowls or glasses, topped with a sprinkle of pumpkin pie spice, a drizzle of maple syrup, or a few pecans for crunch, if desired.

Raw Pecan Pie Bars

Yield: 6 servings | **Prep time:** 20 minutes | **Cook time:** 0 minutes (plus time for chilling)

Ingredients:

For the crust:

- 1 cup raw almonds
- 1 cup pitted dates, soaked in warm water for 10 minutes, then drained
- A pinch of sea salt

For the filling:

- 1 1/2 cups raw pecans, plus more for topping
- 1/2 cup pitted dates, soaked in warm water for 10 minutes, then drained
- 1/4 cup pure maple syrup
- 1 teaspoon vanilla extract
- 1/2 teaspoon ground cinnamon
- A pinch of salt

Nutritional Information: Estimated 350 calories, 6g protein, 45g carbohydrates, 20g fat, 7g fiber, 0mg cholesterol, 50mg sodium, 400mg potassium per serving.

Directions:

1. Prepare the crust: In a food processor, blend the almonds, 1 cup soaked dates, and a pinch of salt until the mixture sticks together when pressed between your fingers. Press the mixture firmly into the bottom of a lined 8x8-inch baking dish.
2. Make the filling: In the same food processor (no need to clean it), blend 1 1/2 cups pecans, 1/2 cup soaked dates, maple syrup, vanilla extract, cinnamon, and a pinch of salt until smooth and spreadable.
3. Spread the pecan filling evenly over the crust. Press additional pecans into the top for decoration, if desired.
4. Chill in the refrigerator for at least 2 hours or until firm. For best results, let it sit overnight.
5. Cut into bars and serve. Store any leftovers in an airtight container in the refrigerator.

Strawberry Basil Ice Pops

Yield: 6 servings | **Prep time:** 15 minutes | **Cook time:** 0 minutes (plus freezing time)

Ingredients:

- 2 cups fresh strawberries, hulled
- 1/4 cup fresh basil leaves
- 3 tablespoons honey or maple syrup
- 1 cup coconut water or plain water

Nutritional Information: Estimated 70 calories, 1g protein, 18g carbohydrates, 0g fat, 2g fiber, 0mg cholesterol, 5mg sodium, 200mg potassium per serving.

Directions:

1. In a blender, combine the strawberries, basil leaves, honey (or maple syrup), and coconut water. Blend until smooth.
2. Taste the mixture and adjust the sweetness if necessary by adding more honey or maple syrup. Blend again if adjustments are made.
3. Pour the mixture into ice pop molds. If your molds have slots for sticks, insert the sticks now. If not, freeze the pops for about 1 hour and then add the sticks when the mixture is semi-frozen.
4. Freeze the ice pops for at least 4 hours or until solid.
5. To serve, run warm water over the outside of the molds for a few seconds to release the ice pops.

Roasted Nut and Cacao Nib Clusters

Yield: 4 servings | **Prep time:** 10 minutes | **Cook time:** 15 minutes

Ingredients:

- 1 cup mixed nuts (such as almonds, walnuts, and pecans)
- 2 tablespoons cacao nibs
- 1 tablespoon coconut oil, melted
- 2 tablespoons honey or maple syrup
- A pinch of sea salt
- 1/2 teaspoon vanilla extract
- Optional: 1/4 teaspoon cinnamon or to taste

Nutritional Information: Estimated 250 calories, 6g protein, 12g carbohydrates, 20g fat, 4g fiber, 0mg cholesterol, 50mg sodium, 300mg potassium per serving.

Directions:

1. Preheat the oven to 350°F (175°C). Line a baking sheet with parchment paper.
2. In a bowl, mix the mixed nuts, cacao nibs, melted coconut oil, honey (or maple syrup), sea salt, vanilla extract, and cinnamon (if using) until well combined.
3. Spread the nut mixture in a single layer on the prepared baking sheet.
4. Roast in the preheated oven for about 12-15 minutes, stirring halfway through, until the nuts are lightly toasted and fragrant.
5. Remove from the oven and allow to cool on the baking sheet. As the mixture cools, it will harden into clusters.
6. Break into clusters once completely cooled. Store in an airtight container at room temperature.

Cherry Almond Clafoutis

Yield: 4 servings | **Prep time:** 15 minutes | **Cook time:** 35 minutes

Ingredients:

- 2 cups fresh cherries, pitted
- 3 large eggs
- 1 cup almond milk
- 1/2 cup almond flour
- 1/4 cup coconut sugar or a suitable substitute
- 1 teaspoon vanilla extract
- 1/2 teaspoon almond extract
- A pinch of salt
- Sliced almonds for garnish
- Optional: A sprinkle of ground cinnamon or nutmeg

Nutritional Information: Estimated 220 calories, 8g protein, 30g carbohydrates, 10g fat, 4g fiber, 140mg cholesterol, 220mg sodium, 350mg potassium per serving.

Directions:

1. Preheat your oven to 350°F (175°C). Lightly grease a 9-inch pie dish or cast iron skillet.
2. Scatter the pitted cherries evenly across the bottom of the prepared dish.
3. In a mixing bowl, whisk together the eggs, almond milk, almond flour, coconut sugar, vanilla extract, almond extract, and a pinch of salt until smooth.
4. Pour the batter over the cherries in the dish. Sprinkle the top with sliced almonds (and a dash of cinnamon or nutmeg, if using).
5. Bake in the preheated oven for 35 minutes, or until the clafoutis is set and golden brown on top. A knife inserted into the center should come out clean.
6. Let cool slightly before serving. It can be enjoyed warm or at room temperature.

Grilled Pineapple with Cinnamon Honey Drizzle

Yield: 4 servings | **Prep time:** 10 minutes | **Cook time:** 10 minutes

Ingredients:

- 1 large pineapple, peeled, cored, and cut into 8 rings
- 1/4 cup honey (preferably raw honey)
- 1 teaspoon ground cinnamon
- A pinch of sea salt
- Cooking spray or olive oil for grilling
- Optional: Fresh mint leaves for garnish

Nutritional Information: Estimated 150 calories, 1g protein, 40g carbohydrates, 0g fat, 2g fiber, 0mg cholesterol, 2mg sodium, 180mg potassium per serving.

Directions:

1. Preheat your grill to medium-high heat. Lightly grease the grill grate with cooking spray or brush with a bit of olive oil to prevent sticking.
2. Mix the honey, ground cinnamon, and a pinch of sea salt in a small bowl. Set aside.
3. Place pineapple rings on the hot grill. Cook for 3-5 minutes on each side or until the pineapple has nice grill marks.
4. Arrange the grilled pineapple rings on a serving platter. Drizzle the cinnamon honey mixture over the warm pineapple.
5. Garnish with fresh mint leaves if desired. Serve immediately.

Fig and Almond Energy Bites

Yield: 20 servings | **Prep time:** 15 minutes | **Cook time:** 0 minutes

Ingredients:

- 1 cup dried figs, stems removed
- 1 cup raw almonds
- 1/2 cup shredded coconut, unsweetened
- 1 tablespoon chia seeds
- 1 tablespoon flaxseed meal
- 1/2 teaspoon ground cinnamon
- 1/4 teaspoon sea salt
- 2 tablespoons coconut oil, melted
- 1 teaspoon vanilla extract

Nutritional Information: Estimated 100 calories, 3g protein, 12g carbohydrates, 6g fat, 3g fiber, 0mg cholesterol, 50mg sodium, 150mg potassium per serving.

Directions:

1. In a food processor, combine the dried figs and almonds. Pulse until coarsely chopped and mixed.
2. Add the shredded coconut, chia seeds, flaxseed meal, ground cinnamon, and sea salt to the food processor. Pulse a few more times until mixed.
3. Pour in the melted coconut oil and vanilla extract. Process until the mixture starts to clump together, forming a sticky dough.
4. Scoop out tablespoon-sized amounts of the mixture and roll into balls. If the mixture is too dry, add a bit of coconut oil or a splash of water to help it stick together.
5. Place the energy bites on a baking sheet lined with parchment paper and refrigerate for at least 30 minutes to set.

Ginger Peach Parfait

Yield: 4 servings | **Prep time:** 15 minutes | **Cook time:** 0 minutes

Ingredients:

- 2 ripe peaches, diced
- 1 tablespoon fresh ginger, grated
- 2 cups Greek yogurt or coconut yogurt (for a vegan option)
- 4 tablespoons honey or maple syrup (for vegan option)
- 1/2 cup granola (ensure gluten-free if necessary)
- 2 tablespoons chia seeds
- Fresh mint leaves for garnish

Nutritional Information: Estimated 200 calories, 10g protein, 30g carbohydrates, 5g fat, 4g fiber, 10mg cholesterol, 50mg sodium, 300mg potassium.

Directions:

1. Mix the diced peaches with the grated ginger and 1 tablespoon of honey or maple syrup in a small bowl. Set aside to marinate for about 10 minutes.
2. Mix the Greek or coconut yogurt with the remaining honey or maple syrup in another bowl.
3. Layer the yogurt mixture, marinated peaches, granola, and chia seeds in serving glasses. Repeat the layers until all ingredients are used.
4. Garnish with fresh mint leaves. Refrigerate for at least 30 minutes before serving to allow the flavors to meld and the chia seeds to slightly swell.
5. Serve chilled.

Chocolate Beetroot Cake

Yield: 4 servings | **Prep time:** 15 minutes | **Cook time:** 45 minutes

Ingredients:

- 1 1/2 cups all-purpose flour (to make it gluten-free, use almond or coconut flour)
- 1/2 cup unsweetened cocoa powder
- 1 cup granulated sugar (or substitute with maple syrup or honey for a natural sweetener)
- 2 tsp baking powder
- 1/2 tsp salt
- 1/3 cup coconut oil, melted
- 1 cup beetroot puree (from cooked and blended beets)
- 2 eggs
- 1 tsp vanilla extract
- 1/2 cup almond milk

Nutritional Information: Estimated 350 calories, 6g protein, 50g carbohydrates, 14g fat, 5g fiber, 55mg cholesterol, 300mg sodium, 400mg potassium.

Directions:

1. Preheat your oven to 350°F (175°C). Grease a 9-inch cake pan and set aside.
2. Whisk together the flour, cocoa powder, sugar, baking powder, and salt in a large mixing bowl.
3. In another bowl, mix the melted coconut oil, beetroot puree, eggs, vanilla extract, and almond milk until well combined.
4. Gradually add the wet ingredients to the dry ingredients, stirring until combined. Avoid overmixing.
5. Pour the batter into the prepared cake pan and smooth the top with a spatula.
6. Bake in the preheated oven for 45 minutes or until a toothpick inserted into the center comes out clean.
7. Let the cake cool in the pan for 10 minutes, then transfer it to a wire rack to cool completely before serving.

Blackberry Mint Frozen Yogurt

Yield: 4 servings | **Prep time:** 10 minutes | **Cook time:** 0 minutes | **Freeze time:** 4 hours

Ingredients:

- 3 cups fresh blackberries
- 2 cups plain Greek yogurt (use dairy-free yogurt for a vegan option)
- 1/4 cup honey or maple syrup (adjust to taste)
- 1 tablespoon fresh mint leaves, finely chopped
- 1 teaspoon vanilla extract

Nutritional Information: Estimated 180 calories, 8g protein, 30g carbohydrates, 2g fat, 5g fiber, 10mg cholesterol, 60mg sodium, 300mg potassium.

Directions:

1. Combine the blackberries, Greek yogurt, honey (or maple syrup), mint leaves, and vanilla extract in a blender. Blend until the mixture is smooth.
2. Taste the mixture and adjust sweetness if necessary, blending again if more honey or maple syrup is added.
3. Pour the mixture into a freezer-safe container. For a smoother texture, stir the mixture every 30 minutes for the first 2 hours of freezing.
4. Freeze until the yogurt is firm, about 4 hours or overnight.
5. Before serving, let the frozen yogurt sit at room temperature for 5-10 minutes to soften slightly for easier scooping.

Snacks

Turmeric Spiced Roasted Chickpeas

Yield: 4 servings | **Prep time:** 10 minutes | **Cook time:** 20 minutes

Ingredients:

- 2 cups cooked chickpeas (or 1 15-oz can, drained and rinsed)
- 1 tablespoon olive oil
- 1 teaspoon ground turmeric
- 1/2 teaspoon garlic powder
- 1/2 teaspoon smoked paprika
- 1/4 teaspoon cayenne pepper (optional, adjust to taste)
- Salt to taste

Nutritional Information: Estimated 134 calories, 4g protein, 18g carbohydrates, 5g fat, 4g fiber, 0mg cholesterol, 200mg sodium, 210mg potassium.

Directions:

1. Preheat your oven to 400°F (200°C). Pat the chickpeas dry with a paper towel to remove any excess moisture. This helps them get crispy.
2. In a bowl, toss the chickpeas with olive oil, turmeric, garlic powder, smoked paprika, cayenne pepper (if using), and salt until evenly coated.
3. Spread the chickpeas in a single layer on a baking sheet lined with parchment paper or a silicone baking mat.
4. Bake for 20 minutes or until crispy and golden brown. Shake the pan or stir the chickpeas halfway through to ensure even roasting.
5. Let cool before serving. They will continue to crisp up as they cool.

Kale Chips with Nutritional Yeast

Yield: 4 servings | **Prep time:** 10 minutes | **Cook time:** 20 minutes

Ingredients:

- 1 large bunch of kale, stems removed and leaves torn into bite-sized pieces
- 1 tablespoon olive oil
- 2 tablespoons nutritional yeast
- 1/2 teaspoon garlic powder
- 1/4 teaspoon salt
- 1/4 teaspoon black pepper

Nutritional Information: Estimated 58 calories, 4g protein, 7g carbohydrates, 3g fat, 2g fiber, 0mg cholesterol, 150mg sodium, 300mg potassium.

Directions:

1. Preheat your oven to 300°F (150°C). Line a baking sheet with parchment paper.
2. Toss the kale pieces with olive oil in a large bowl, ensuring each piece is lightly coated. Sprinkle nutritional yeast, garlic powder, salt, and pepper over the kale and toss again to distribute the seasoning evenly.
3. Arrange the kale in a single layer on the prepared baking sheet, ensuring the pieces don't overlap to allow for even baking.
4. Bake for 20 minutes or until the kale chips are crispy and lightly browned at the edges. Check halfway through and stir if necessary to ensure even baking.
5. Remove from oven and let cool for a few minutes before serving. The chips will continue to crisp up as they cool.

Almond Butter and Banana on Sprouted Grain Toast

Yield: 2 servings | **Prep time:** 5 minutes | **Cook time:** 2 minutes

Ingredients:

- 2 slices of sprouted grain bread (or gluten-free)
- 4 tablespoons almond butter
- 1 medium banana, sliced
- A pinch of ground cinnamon (optional)
- A drizzle of honey (optional)

Nutritional Information: Estimated 350 calories, 10g protein, 45g carbohydrates, 18g fat, 8g fiber, 0mg cholesterol, 200mg sodium, 450mg potassium.

Directions:

1. Toast the sprouted grain bread slices to your desired level of crispiness.
2. Spread 2 tablespoons of almond butter evenly over each slice of toast.
3. Arrange banana slices over the almond butter on each toast. Sprinkle a pinch of ground cinnamon and drizzle honey over the top for added sweetness and flavor.
4. Serve immediately for a satisfying and nutritious breakfast or snack.

Beetroot Hummus with Cucumber Sticks

Yield: 4 servings | **Prep time:** 10 minutes | **Cook time:** 0 minutes

Ingredients:

- 1 medium beetroot, cooked and peeled
- 1 can (15 oz) chickpeas, drained and rinsed
- 2 tablespoons tahini
- 2 cloves garlic, minced
- Juice of 1 lemon
- 2 tablespoons extra virgin olive oil
- Salt and pepper, to taste
- 1 large cucumber, cut into sticks

Nutritional Information: Estimated 200 calories, 6g protein, 22g carbohydrates, 10g fat, 6g fiber, 0mg cholesterol, 300mg sodium, 400mg potassium.

Directions:

1. Blend the cooked beetroot, chickpeas, tahini, garlic, lemon juice, and olive oil until smooth in a food processor. Season with salt and pepper to taste.
2. Transfer the hummus to a serving bowl. If desired, drizzle with more olive oil and a sprinkle of sesame seeds for garnish.
3. Serve the beetroot hummus with cucumber sticks for dipping.
4. For an extra touch, garnish with chopped parsley or cilantro.
5. Store any leftover hummus in an airtight container in the refrigerator for up to 5 days.

Spicy Pumpkin Seeds

Yield: 4 servings | **Prep time:** 10 minutes | **Cook time:** 15 minutes

Ingredients:

- 1 cup raw pumpkin seeds, cleaned and dried
- 1 tablespoon olive oil
- 1/2 teaspoon ground cumin
- 1/4 teaspoon cayenne pepper (adjust according to spice preference)
- 1/2 teaspoon smoked paprika
- 1/4 teaspoon garlic powder
- Salt to taste

Nutritional Information: Estimated 180 calories, 9g protein, 3g carbohydrates, 15g fat, 2g fiber, 0mg cholesterol, 120mg sodium, 260mg potassium.

Directions:

1. Preheat your oven to 375°F (190°C) and line a baking sheet with parchment paper.
2. Toss the pumpkin seeds with olive oil, cumin, cayenne pepper, smoked paprika, garlic powder, and salt until well coated.
3. Spread the seasoned pumpkin seeds in a single layer on the prepared baking sheet.
4. Bake in the preheated oven for about 15 minutes or until the seeds are golden and crispy, stirring halfway through to ensure even cooking.
5. Let cool before serving. Pumpkin seeds can be stored in an airtight container for up to a week.

Baked Apple Chips with Cinnamon

Yield: 4 servings | **Prep time:** 10 minutes | **Cook time:** 2 hours

Ingredients:

- 2 large apples, any sweet variety
- 1 teaspoon ground cinnamon
- 1/4 teaspoon ground nutmeg (optional)
- A sprinkle of sea salt

Nutritional Information: Estimated 95 calories, 0.5g protein, 25g carbohydrates, 0.3g fat, 4.5g fiber, 0mg cholesterol, 2mg sodium, 195mg potassium.

Directions:

1. Preheat your oven to 200°F (93°C). Line two baking sheets with parchment paper.
2. Core the apples and thinly slice them to about 1/8 inch thick. A mandoline slicer works best for uniform thin slices.
3. In a large bowl, gently toss the apple slices with cinnamon, nutmeg (if using), and a light sprinkle of sea salt until evenly coated.
4. Arrange the apple slices in a single layer on the prepared baking sheets. Ensure they do not overlap to promote even drying.
5. Bake for 1 hour, flip the slices, and continue baking for another 1 hour or until the apple slices are dry and crispy. Baking time may vary based on the oven and the thickness of the slices.
6. Let the apple chips cool completely on the baking sheet. They will continue to crisp up as they cool.

Sweet Potato and Avocado Bites

Yield: 4 servings | **Prep time:** 15 minutes | **Cook time:** 25 minutes

Ingredients:

- 2 large sweet potatoes, peeled and cut into 1/2-inch thick rounds
- 2 tablespoons olive oil
- Salt and pepper, to taste
- 1 ripe avocado
- Juice of 1 lime
- 1/4 teaspoon garlic powder
- 1/4 teaspoon chili powder (optional)
- Fresh cilantro for garnish
- Crushed red pepper flakes for garnish (optional)

Nutritional Information: Estimated 200 calories, 3g protein, 24g carbohydrates, 11g fat, 7g fiber, 0mg cholesterol, 120mg sodium, 670mg potassium.

Directions:

1. Preheat your oven to 400°F (200°C). Line a baking sheet with parchment paper.
2. Toss the sweet potato rounds with olive oil, salt, and pepper. Arrange them in a single layer on the baking sheet.
3. Bake for 20-25 minutes or until tender and slightly golden, flipping halfway through.
4. While the sweet potatoes are baking, mash the avocado in a bowl. Stir in the lime juice, garlic powder, chili powder (if using), and season with salt and pepper to taste.
5. Once the sweet potato rounds are done, let them cool slightly. Top each round with a dollop of the avocado mixture.
6. Garnish with fresh cilantro and red pepper flakes (if desired) before serving.

Almond and Date Energy Balls

Yield: 4 servings | **Prep time:** 10 minutes | **Cook time:** 0 minutes

Ingredients:

- 1 cup almonds
- 1 cup dates, pitted
- 1/4 cup unsweetened shredded coconut
- 1 tablespoon chia seeds
- 1 tablespoon flaxseed meal
- 2 tablespoons coconut oil
- 1 teaspoon vanilla extract
- A pinch of salt

Nutritional Information: Estimated 300 calories, 6g protein, 24g carbohydrates, 22g fat, 7g fiber, 0mg cholesterol, 50mg sodium, 350mg potassium.

Directions:

1. Place almonds in a food processor and pulse until coarsely ground.
2. Add the dates, shredded coconut, chia seeds, flaxseed meal, coconut oil, vanilla extract, and a pinch of salt. Process until the mixture sticks together when pressed between your fingers.
3. Scoop out tablespoon-sized amounts of the mixture and roll into balls.
4. Place the energy balls on a baking sheet lined with parchment paper and refrigerate for at least 30 minutes to set.
5. Store in an airtight container in the refrigerator for up to a week or freeze for extended storage.

Coconut Yogurt Parfait with Mixed Berries

Yield: 4 servings | **Prep time:** 10 minutes | **Cook time:** 0 minutes

Ingredients:

- 2 cups unsweetened coconut yogurt
- 1 cup mixed berries (blueberries, raspberries, strawberries)
- 1/4 cup granola (ensure gluten-free if necessary for an anti-inflammatory diet)
- 2 tablespoons chia seeds
- 2 tablespoons honey or maple syrup (optional for sweetness)
- A handful of fresh mint leaves for garnish

Nutritional Information: Estimated 220 calories, 5g protein, 25g carbohydrates, 12g fat, 6g fiber, 0mg cholesterol, 30mg sodium, 200mg potassium.

Directions:

1. In four glasses or parfait cups, layer 1/4 cup of coconut yogurt at the bottom of each.
2. Add a layer of mixed berries on top of the yogurt.
3. Sprinkle a tablespoon of granola over the berries, then add a layer of chia seeds.
4. Repeat the layering process until all ingredients are used up, finishing with a layer of berries on top.
5. Drizzle with some honey or maple syrup for added sweetness, if desired.
6. Garnish with fresh mint leaves before serving.

Flaxseed and Walnut Crackers

Yield: 4 servings | **Prep time:** 15 minutes | **Cook time:** 30 minutes

Ingredients:

- 1 cup ground flaxseeds
- 1/2 cup finely chopped walnuts
- 2 tablespoons chia seeds
- 1 cup water
- 1/2 teaspoon sea salt
- 1/4 teaspoon garlic powder
- 1/4 teaspoon onion powder

Nutritional Information: Estimated 200 calories, 6g protein, 10g carbohydrates, 15g fat, 8g fiber, 0mg cholesterol, 150mg sodium, 300mg potassium.

Directions:

1. Preheat your oven to 350°F (175°C) and line a baking sheet with parchment paper.
2. Mix the ground flaxseeds, chopped walnuts, chia seeds, sea salt, garlic powder, and onion powder in a large bowl.
3. Add water to the dry ingredients and stir until well combined. Let the mixture sit for about 5 minutes to thicken.
4. Spread the mixture evenly onto the prepared baking sheet, aiming for about 1/4 inch thickness.
5. Bake in the preheated oven for 30 minutes or until the edges are crispy and the center is firm.
6. Remove from the oven and let cool completely before breaking into pieces.

Broccoli and Cauliflower Buffalo Bites

Yield: 4 servings | **Prep time:** 15 minutes | **Cook time:** 25 minutes

Ingredients:

- 2 cups broccoli florets
- 2 cups cauliflower florets
- 1 cup almond flour
- 1 cup unsweetened almond milk
- 1/2 cup buffalo sauce
- 1 teaspoon garlic powder
- 1 teaspoon paprika
- Salt and pepper to taste
- Optional: Fresh parsley for garnish

Nutritional Information: Estimated 250 calories, 8g protein, 18g carbohydrates, 16g fat, 6g fiber, 0mg cholesterol, 500mg sodium, 350mg potassium.

Directions:

1. Preheat the oven to 425°F (220°C) and line a baking sheet with parchment paper.
2. Whisk together the almond flour, almond milk, garlic powder, paprika, salt, and pepper in a large bowl until smooth.
3. Dip the broccoli and cauliflower florets into the batter, ensuring each piece is well-coated. Place the coated florets on the prepared baking sheet in a single layer.
4. Bake for 20 minutes, flipping halfway through, until the coating is golden and crispy.
5. Remove the florets from the oven and gently toss them with buffalo sauce. Return to the oven and bake for an additional 5 minutes.
6. Garnish with fresh parsley, if desired, and serve immediately.

Pineapple and Ginger Smoothie

Yield: 2 servings | **Prep time:** 10 minutes | **Cook time:** 0 minutes

Ingredients:

- 2 cups fresh pineapple chunks
- 1-inch fresh ginger, peeled and grated
- 1 cup unsweetened almond milk
- 1/2 cup coconut water
- 1 tablespoon chia seeds
- 1 tablespoon honey (optional; adjust based on dietary needs)
- Ice cubes (optional)

Nutritional Information: Estimated 150 calories, 3g protein, 28g carbohydrates, 2g fat, 4g fiber, 0mg cholesterol, 50mg sodium, 400mg potassium.

Directions:

1. In a blender, combine the pineapple chunks, grated ginger, almond milk, coconut water, chia seeds, and honey (if using). Add ice cubes if you prefer a colder smoothie.
2. Blend on high speed until smooth and creamy. If the smoothie is too thick, add more coconut water or almond milk to reach your desired consistency.
3. Taste and adjust the sweetness by adding more honey if necessary.
4. Pour into glasses and serve immediately.

Cashew Turmeric Latte

Yield: 2 servings | **Prep time:** 5 minutes | **Cook time:** 5 minutes

Ingredients:

- 1 cup raw cashews, soaked overnight and drained
- 2 cups water
- 1 tablespoon turmeric powder
- 1 teaspoon cinnamon
- 1/4 teaspoon ground ginger
- 2 tablespoons maple syrup or honey (optional for sweetness)
- Pinch of black pepper (to activate turmeric's benefits)
- 1 teaspoon vanilla extract

Nutritional Information: Nutritional values for this recipe will vary based on specific ingredient choices and portion sizes. You can use a healthy calculator online to input the ingredients and quantities to calculate precise dietary information. This will provide the calories, protein, carbohydrates, fat, fiber, cholesterol, sodium, and potassium values.

Directions:

1. In a high-speed blender, blend soaked and drained cashews with water until smooth to make cashew milk.
2. Pour the cashew milk into a saucepan and add turmeric, cinnamon, ground ginger, maple syrup (if using), black pepper, and vanilla extract.
3. Heat the mixture over medium heat for about 5 minutes or until warm but not boiling. Stir frequently to ensure the spices are well incorporated.
4. Taste and adjust sweetness if necessary.
5. Serve warm in mugs. Optionally, you can froth the top with a milk frother for a latte effect.

Avocado and Tomato Salsa Cups

Yield: 4 servings | **Prep time:** 20 minutes | **Cook time:** 0 minutes

Ingredients:

- 2 ripe avocados, peeled, pitted, and diced
- 1 large tomato, diced
- 1/4 cup red onion, finely chopped
- 2 tablespoons cilantro, chopped
- 1 lime, juiced
- Salt and pepper to taste
- 1 jalapeno, seeded and finely chopped (optional)
- 8 small lettuce leaves (such as Bibb or Romaine) for serving

Nutritional Information: Estimated 170 calories, 2g protein, 10g carbohydrates, 15g fat, 7g fiber, 0mg cholesterol, 10mg sodium, 500mg potassium.

Directions:

1. Gently mix the avocados, tomato, red onion, cilantro, lime juice, and jalapeno in a medium bowl. Season with salt and pepper to taste.
2. Carefully spoon the mixture into the lettuce leaves, dividing evenly.
3. Serve immediately or chill in the refrigerator for up to an hour before serving to let the flavors meld.

Spiced Roasted Nuts with Rosemary

Yield: 4 servings | **Prep time:** 10 minutes | **Cook time:** 20 minutes

Ingredients:

- 2 cups mixed nuts (such as almonds, walnuts, and pecans)
- 1 tablespoon olive oil
- 2 tablespoons fresh rosemary, finely chopped
- 1 teaspoon sea salt
- 1/2 teaspoon ground black pepper
- 1/4 teaspoon cayenne pepper
- 1 tablespoon brown sugar
- 1/2 teaspoon garlic powder

Nutritional Information: Estimated 400 calories, 10g protein, 20g carbohydrates, 3g fat, 5g fiber, 0mg cholesterol, 300mg sodium, 450mg potassium.

Directions:

1. Preheat your oven to 350°F (175°C). Combine the mixed nuts with olive oil in a large bowl, ensuring all the nuts are evenly coated.
2. Add the chopped rosemary, sea salt, black pepper, cayenne pepper, brown sugar, and garlic powder to the nuts. Toss well to ensure the nuts are evenly coated with the spice mixture.
3. Spread the nuts in a single layer on a baking sheet lined with parchment paper. Bake in the preheated oven for 20 minutes, stirring halfway through the cooking time to ensure even roasting.
4. Remove the nuts from the oven and let them cool on the baking sheet. They will become crunchier as they cool.

Sweet Potato Toast with Almond Butter

Yield: 4 servings | **Prep time:** 5 minutes | **Cook time:** 15 minutes

Ingredients:

- 2 large sweet potatoes, sliced lengthwise into 1/4-inch thick slices
- 1/2 cup almond butter
- Optional toppings: sliced bananas, chia seeds, honey, or berries

Nutritional Information: Estimated 280 calories, 8g protein, 33g carbohydrates, 14g fat, 6g fiber, 0mg cholesterol, 100mg sodium, 440mg potassium.

Directions:

1. Preheat your oven to 400°F (200°C). Arrange the sweet potato slices in a single layer on a baking sheet lined with parchment paper.
2. Bake in the preheated oven for about 15 minutes or until the slices are tender and slightly crispy at the edges. Alternatively, you can toast the sweet potato slices in a toaster on the highest setting for two cycles or until they are cooked through and slightly crispy.
3. Spread almond butter over each sweet potato slice. If desired, top with your choice of sliced bananas, chia seeds, honey, or berries for extra flavor and nutrients.
4. Serve immediately as a healthy and filling breakfast or snack option.

Mango and Avocado Salsa with Homemade Plantain Chips

Yield: 4 servings | **Prep time:** 20 minutes | **Cook time:** 20 minutes

Ingredients:

For the Salsa:

- 1 ripe mango, peeled and diced
- 1 ripe avocado, peeled and diced
- 1/2 red onion, finely chopped
- 1/4 cup fresh cilantro, chopped
- Juice of 1 lime
- Salt and pepper to taste

For the Plantain Chips:

- 2 green plantains
- 1/4 cup olive oil
- Salt to taste

Nutritional Information: Estimated 320 calories, 2g protein, 45g carbohydrates, 16g fat, 7g fiber, 0mg cholesterol, 150mg sodium, 700mg potassium.

Directions:

1. Preheat the oven to 350°F (175°C). Peel the plantains and slice them thinly using a mandoline slicer or a sharp knife. Toss the slices with olive oil and a pinch of salt, ensuring each slice is well coated.
2. Arrange the plantain slices in a single layer on a baking sheet lined with parchment paper. Bake for 15-20 minutes, flipping halfway through, until they are crispy and golden. Remove from the oven and let them cool.
3. While the plantain chips are baking, prepare the salsa. Combine diced mango, avocado, red onion, cilantro, and lime juice in a mixing bowl. Season with salt and pepper to taste. Gently toss to mix without mashing the avocado.
4. For dipping, serve the mango and avocado salsa with the homemade plantain chips on the side.

Lemon and Herb Marinated Olives

Yield: 4 servings | **Prep time:** 10 minutes | **Cook time:** 0 minutes

Ingredients:

- 2 cups mixed olives, drained
- Zest 1 lemon in strips
- 2 tablespoons lemon juice
- 2 cloves garlic, thinly sliced
- 2 tablespoons extra virgin olive oil
- 1 tablespoon fresh rosemary, chopped
- 1 tablespoon fresh thyme, chopped
- 1/4 teaspoon red pepper flakes (optional)

Nutritional Information: Estimated 150 calories, 1g protein, 4g carbohydrates, 15g fat, 2g fiber, 0mg cholesterol, 800mg sodium (varies depending on the sodium content of the olives used), 50mg potassium.

Directions:

1. Combine the mixed olives, lemon zest strips, lemon juice, sliced garlic, extra virgin olive oil, chopped rosemary, chopped thyme, and red pepper flakes in a medium bowl. Mix well to ensure the olives are evenly coated with the marinade.
2. Cover the bowl with plastic wrap or transfer the mixture to a jar with a tight-fitting lid. Refrigerate for at least 2 hours or overnight for the flavors to meld. The longer the olives marinate, the more pronounced the flavors will be.
3. Before serving, let the olives come to room temperature to ensure the olive oil returns to a liquid state and the flavors are more pronounced.
4. Serve as a part of an appetizer spread or as a flavorful addition to salads.

Pumpkin Spice Roasted Almonds

Yield: 4 servings | **Prep time:** 5 minutes | **Cook time:** 20 minutes

Ingredients:

- 2 cups raw almonds
- 1 tablespoon olive oil
- 2 tablespoons maple syrup
- 1 teaspoon ground cinnamon
- 1/2 teaspoon ground nutmeg
- 1/2 teaspoon ground ginger
- 1/4 teaspoon ground cloves
- 1/4 teaspoon salt

Nutritional Information: Estimated 350 calories, 12g protein, 20g carbohydrates, 28g fat, 6g fiber, 0mg cholesterol, 150mg sodium, 400mg potassium.

Directions:

1. Preheat your oven to 325°F (165°C). Mix the almonds with olive oil and maple syrup in a large bowl until they are evenly coated.
2. Combine the cinnamon, nutmeg, ginger, cloves, and salt in a small bowl. Sprinkle the spice mixture over the almonds and toss until the almonds are evenly coated with the spices.
3. Spread the almonds in a single layer on a baking sheet lined with parchment paper. Bake in the preheated oven for 20 minutes, stirring once halfway through to ensure even roasting.
4. Remove the almonds from the oven and let them cool on the baking sheet. They will become crunchier as they cool.

Avocado Lime Hummus

Yield: 4 servings | **Prep time:** 10 minutes | **Cook time:** 0 minutes

Ingredients:

- 1 (15 oz) can chickpeas, drained and rinsed
- 1 ripe avocado, peeled and pitted
- 2 tablespoons tahini
- 2 tablespoons olive oil
- Juice of 1 lime (about 2 tablespoons)
- 1 clove garlic, minced
- 1/2 teaspoon salt
- 1/4 teaspoon ground cumin
- 2-4 tablespoons water (as needed for desired consistency)
- Fresh cilantro for garnish (optional)

Nutritional Information: Estimated 250 calories, 7g protein, 20g carbohydrates, 17g fat, 7g fiber, 0mg cholesterol, 300mg sodium, 400mg potassium.

Directions:

1. In the bowl of a food processor, combine the chickpeas, avocado, tahini, olive oil, lime juice, garlic, salt, and cumin. Process until smooth.
2. While the food processor is running, slowly add water, one tablespoon at a time, until the hummus reaches your desired consistency.
3. Taste and adjust seasoning if necessary. For a more pronounced lime flavor, you may add additional lime juice.
4. Transfer the hummus to a serving bowl and garnish with fresh cilantro if desired. Serve immediately with your choice of vegetables or pita chips, or use as a spread for sandwiches.

Part 4: Lifestyle Changes for Reducing Inflammation

Incorporating Physical Activity: The Importance of Regular Exercise in Reducing Inflammation

Embarking on an anti-inflammatory diet is a transformative step toward better health, but the journey doesn't stop at the dinner table. Incorporating regular physical activity into your lifestyle is essential to combat inflammation and enhance your overall wellness. This chapter explores the symbiotic relationship between exercise and an anti-inflammatory diet, offering beginners practical advice on integrating physical activity to reduce inflammation.

The Link Between Exercise and Inflammation

Physical activity is a powerful ally in the fight against inflammation. Regular exercise helps reduce inflammatory markers, such as C-reactive protein (CRP) and tumor necrosis factor-alpha (TNF-alpha), often elevated in chronic inflammatory conditions. Furthermore, exercise promotes the release of anti-inflammatory substances by the body, helping to counteract inflammation from within.

Types of Exercise to Combat Inflammation

Not all exercise is created equal when it comes to fighting inflammation. A balanced approach that includes a variety of activities can offer the most benefits:

- Aerobic Exercise: Activities like walking, cycling, swimming, and jogging improve cardiovascular health and help lower fat levels, reducing inflammatory markers.
- Strength Training: Building muscle through resistance training can help regulate blood sugar levels and decrease fat, which is essential for reducing inflammation.
- Flexibility and Balance Exercises: Practices such as yoga and tai chi enhance flexibility and balance and reduce stress levels, which is crucial since stress can exacerbate inflammation.

Starting Your Exercise Journey

Incorporating exercise into a daily routine can take time and effort for beginners. Here are some tips to get started:

- Set Realistic Goals: Begin with small, achievable goals, such as a 10-minute walk each day, gradually increasing the duration and intensity as your fitness improves.
- Find Activities You Enjoy: Exercise doesn't have to be a chore. Whether dancing, hiking, or playing a sport, engaging in activities you love can make exercise something to look forward to.

- Listen to Your Body: Starting an exercise routine can be challenging. Pay attention to your body's signals and adjust your activities to avoid overexertion, which can lead to increased inflammation.

The Role of Recovery

Recovery is as important as the exercise itself. Adequate rest, including good sleep quality and rest days, allows the body to heal and repair, preventing the onset of inflammation due to overtraining. Incorporating anti-inflammatory foods into your post-workout meals can enhance recovery and reduce inflammation.

Incorporating Physical Activity Into Your Anti-Inflammatory Lifestyle

Aim to integrate physical activity into your daily routine to maximize the benefits of an anti-inflammatory diet. This doesn't mean you need to spend hours at the gym; even simple changes like taking the stairs instead of the elevator, engaging in active play with children or pets, or opting for a walking meeting can increase your activity levels.

Stress Management Techniques: Mitigating Stress to Combat Inflammation

While diet and exercise are critical components of managing inflammation, the role of psychological well-being cannot be overstated. Physical and emotional stress plays a significant part in exacerbating inflammatory responses within the body. This chapter delves into the intricate relationship between stress and inflammation and outlines practical strategies for stress management, an essential aspect of an anti-inflammatory lifestyle.

Understanding the Stress-Inflammation Connection

The body's stress response, often called "fight or flight," is designed to protect us in times of danger. However, in our modern lifestyle, chronic stress triggers this response continuously, leading to elevated levels of cortisol and other stress hormones. These hormones can disrupt immune system function and exacerbate inflammation, contributing to various chronic diseases.

Identifying Stressors

The first step in managing stress is recognizing its sources. Stressors can be external, like work pressure, relationship issues, or internal, stemming from chronic worry or negative thought patterns. Identifying what triggers your stress is crucial in developing effective coping mechanisms.

Stress Management Techniques

Implementing stress reduction techniques can significantly lower inflammation levels. Here are some strategies to incorporate into your anti-inflammatory lifestyle:

- Mindfulness and Meditation: Mindfulness meditation, deep breathing exercises, and progressive muscle relaxation can help calm the mind and reduce the body's stress response.
- Physical Activity: Regular exercise is not only good for physical health but also for mental well-being.
- Adequate Sleep: Poor sleep can exacerbate stress and inflammation. Establishing a regular sleep schedule and creating a restful environment can improve sleep quality.
- Healthy Social Connections: Spending time with friends and family or engaging in community activities can provide emotional support and reduce stress.
- Time Management: Overcommitment can lead to stress. Learning to say no and prioritizing your tasks can help manage your workload and reduce stress.
- Connecting with Nature: Time spent in natural environments can lower stress levels and, by extension, inflammation.
- Nutrition: Certain foods can have a calming effect on the body. Incorporating anti-inflammatory foods rich in omega-3 fatty acids, antioxidants, and fiber can support your body's ability to handle stress.

Integrating Stress Management into Your Lifestyle

Adopting a holistic approach to stress management involves integrating these techniques into your daily routine. It might mean setting aside time for meditation, prioritizing physical activity, ensuring enough rest, or making dietary adjustments. The key is consistency and making these practices a regular part of your lifestyle.

Sleep Hygiene: Enhancing Sleep to Reduce Inflammation

In the quest for a healthier, anti-inflammatory lifestyle, sleep plays a pivotal role that is often underestimated. Sleep quality directly impacts your body's inflammatory processes, making sleep hygiene—an array of practices that promote regular, restful sleep—a cornerstone of managing inflammation. This chapter explores the critical relationship between sleep and inflammation and offers practical advice for improving sleep quality.

The Sleep-Inflammation Connection

Research has consistently shown that inadequate sleep—whether in duration or quality—can lead to increased levels of inflammatory markers in the body. This elevation is linked to a higher risk of developing chronic diseases such as heart disease, diabetes, and obesity, all of which have inflammation as a common underlying factor. Furthermore, poor sleep can exacerbate existing inflammatory conditions, creating a cycle of inflammation and sleep disturbances.

Recognizing Sleep Disruptors

Various factors can impair your ability to get a good night's sleep, including stress, poor diet, lack of physical activity, and an unsuitable sleep environment. Identifying and addressing these disruptors is the first step toward improving sleep hygiene.

Strategies for Improved Sleep Hygiene

Improving your sleep quality can have a profound impact on reducing inflammation. Here are some strategies to enhance your sleep hygiene:

- Establish a Consistent Sleep Schedule: Going to bed and waking up at the same time each day, even on weekends, helps regulate your body's internal clock and improves sleep quality.
- Create a Restful Environment: Ensure your bedroom is conducive to sleep—relaxed, quiet, and dark. Investing in a comfortable mattress and pillows can also make a significant difference.
- Limit Exposure to Screens Before Bed: The blue light emitted by phones, tablets, and computers can interfere with your ability to fall asleep. Try to avoid screens for at least an hour before bedtime.
- Incorporate Relaxation Techniques: Practices like reading, meditating, or taking a warm bath before bed can help signal your body that it's time to wind down.
- Watch Your Diet: Avoid heavy meals, caffeine, and alcohol close to bedtime, as they can disrupt sleep. Instead, focus on foods that promote sleep, such as those rich in magnesium and tryptophan.
- Exercise Regularly: Regular physical activity can help you fall asleep faster and enjoy deeper sleep. However, try not to exercise too close to bedtime, as it can be stimulating.
- Manage Stress: Stress and worry can lead to insomnia. Techniques such as journaling, mindfulness, and deep breathing exercises can help manage stress levels before bed.

The Role of Diet in Sleep

An anti-inflammatory diet not only helps reduce inflammation but can also improve sleep quality. Foods rich in omega-3 fatty acids, magnesium, and antioxidants can support better sleep. Cherries, for example, are a natural source of melatonin, while fatty fish like salmon provide omega-3s that have been shown to improve sleep quality.

Tracking Your Progress: Monitoring Changes with an Anti-Inflammatory Lifestyle

Adopting an anti-inflammatory diet is a transformative journey toward improved health and well-being. However, understanding and tracking the impact of these dietary changes on your body is crucial for maintaining motivation and making necessary adjustments. This chapter provides practical tips on monitoring changes in health markers, symptoms, and overall well-being as you embrace an anti-inflammatory lifestyle.

Setting Baselines

Before you begin your anti-inflammatory journey, it's essential to establish baselines for various health markers and symptoms. This might include:

- Inflammatory markers: Consider getting a blood test to measure levels of inflammatory markers such as C-reactive protein (CRP), which can provide insight into your body's baseline level of inflammation.
- Symptoms: List any symptoms you're experiencing, such as joint pain, fatigue, or gastrointestinal issues. Rate their severity on a scale from 1 to 10.
- Weight and Body Measurements: While not directly related to inflammation, changes in weight and body measurements can reflect improvements in overall health.
- Energy Levels and Mood: Note your general energy levels and mood, as improvements in diet can often lead to enhanced well-being in these areas.

Monitoring Dietary Changes

Keep a food diary to track what you eat and drink, focusing on incorporating anti-inflammatory foods and eliminating or reducing inflammatory ones. Note any new foods you introduce to your diet and how you feel after consuming them. This can help identify foods that particularly benefit you or may still trigger inflammation or discomfort.

Tracking Symptom Changes

Regularly update the list of symptoms you established at the beginning of your journey, noting any changes in their frequency and severity. Improvements in these symptoms can be a strong indicator of the benefits your dietary changes are providing.

Observing Changes in Health Markers

If possible, schedule follow-up blood tests to measure inflammatory markers after several months of following an anti-inflammatory diet. Comparing these results with your baseline can offer objective evidence of the diet's impact on your health.

Assessing Energy Levels and Mood

Reflect on your energy levels and mood as you progress with your anti-inflammatory lifestyle. Many individuals notice improvements in these areas as their diet becomes more prosperous in nutrients that support overall health and reduce inflammation.

Using Technology and Resources

Consider utilizing apps and tools designed for health tracking. Many apps allow you to log food intake, symptoms, and activity levels, making it easier to spot trends and correlations over time.

Reflecting on Your Journey

Regularly review your progress, not just in terms of physical health but also in your relationship with food and your overall lifestyle. Celebrate successes, no matter how small, and consider any setbacks as opportunities to learn and adjust your approach.

Part 5: Meal Plan and Shopping List

Embarking on an anti-inflammatory diet can be both an exciting and daunting journey. In Part 5 of our cookbook, we've meticulously crafted a comprehensive 30-day meal plan to ease beginners into anti-inflammatory eating. This chapter outlines daily meals that are delicious and simple to prepare and emphasizes variety and nutritional balance. From the vibrant Golden Turmeric Porridge to the hearty Sweet Potato and Black Bean Chili, each recipe has been chosen for its health benefits and flavor.

To streamline your transition, we've also compiled an exhaustive shopping list that categorizes ingredients into fruits, vegetables, proteins, grains, and more, ensuring you have everything you need to begin your journey toward reduced inflammation and improved overall health. This list reflects the diversity of ingredients used throughout the meal plan, highlighting the importance of whole, nutrient-dense foods in combating inflammation.

Whether you're entirely new to the concept or looking to refine your approach to an anti-inflammatory diet, this chapter serves as your roadmap. It's designed to remove the guesswork from meal planning and grocery shopping, allowing you to focus on the enjoyment and satisfaction of nourishing your body with the best foods nature offers.

30 days meal plan

Week 1

Day 1:

- **Breakfast:** Golden Turmeric Porridge
- **Lunch:** Quinoa Salad with Chickpeas and Avocado
- **Dinner:** Turmeric Ginger Grilled Chicken

Day 2:

- **Breakfast:** Chia and Hemp Seed Superfood Pudding
- **Lunch:** Grilled Chicken and Roasted Vegetable Bowl
- **Dinner:** Baked Salmon with Walnut Pesto

Day 3:

- **Breakfast:** Avocado and Egg Breakfast Bowl
- **Lunch:** Lentil Soup with Kale and Sweet Potatoes
- **Dinner:** Sweet Potato and Black Bean Chili

Day 4:

- **Breakfast:** Ginger Infused Mixed Berry Smoothie
- **Lunch:** Vegan Black Bean and Quinoa Stuffed Peppers
- **Dinner:** Cauliflower Steak with Tahini Sauce

Day 5:

- **Breakfast:** Cinnamon Spiced Baked Apples with Walnuts
- **Lunch:** Baked Tofu and Vegetable Stir-Fry over Whole Grain Noodles
- **Dinner:** Moroccan Vegetable Tagine

Day 6:

- **Breakfast:** Quinoa Breakfast Muffins
- **Lunch:** Spicy Sweet Potato and Black Bean Burrito Bowl
- **Dinner:** Mediterranean Chickpea Salad

Day 7:

- **Breakfast:** Sweet Potato and Kale Hash with Poached Eggs
- **Lunch:** Grilled Vegetable and Hummus Wraps
- **Dinner:** Stuffed Bell Peppers with Quinoa and Spinach

Week 2

Day 8:

- **Breakfast:** Flaxseed and Banana Pancakes
- **Lunch:** Cauliflower Rice Tabbouleh with Grilled Chicken
- **Dinner:** Quinoa Tabbouleh with Lemon Mint Dressing

Day 9:

- **Breakfast:** Spinach, Feta, and Red Pepper Omelette
- **Lunch:** Spinach, Walnut, and Strawberry Salad with Grilled Shrimp
- **Dinner:** Broccoli and Almond Stir-Fry

Day 10:

- **Breakfast:** Coconut Yogurt with Pomegranate and Almonds
- **Lunch:** Zucchini Noodles with Avocado Pesto and Cherry Tomatoes
- **Dinner:** Grilled Eggplant with Herbed Quinoa

Day 11:

- **Breakfast:** Carrot and Ginger Warm Breakfast Salad
- **Lunch:** Moroccan Lentil and Vegetable Stew
- **Dinner:** Butternut Squash Soup with Coconut Milk

Day 12:

- **Breakfast:** Broccoli and Quinoa Breakfast Casserole
- **Lunch:** Beetroot, Goat Cheese, and Arugula Salad with Roasted Beets
- **Dinner:** Wild Salmon with Sautéed Spinach and Mushrooms

Day 13:

- **Breakfast:** Pumpkin Spice Chia Seed Pudding
- **Lunch:** Soba Noodles with Edamame and Cucumber
- **Dinner:** Vegan Lentil Bolognese with Zoodles

Day 14:

- **Breakfast:** Savory Turmeric and Black Pepper Oats with Avocado
- **Lunch:** Cold Quinoa Salad with Lemon Herb Dressing
- **Dinner:** Thai Coconut Curry with Tofu

Week 3

Day 15:

- **Breakfast:** Zucchini Bread with Flaxseeds
- **Lunch:** Vegan Buddha Bowl with Tahini Dressing
- **Dinner:** Lemon Herb Roasted Chicken with Asparagus

Day 16:

- **Breakfast:** Buckwheat Pancakes with Mixed Berry Compote
- **Lunch:** Shrimp and Mango Salad with Citrus Vinaigrette
- **Dinner:** Vegan Mushroom Stroganoff

Day 17:

- **Breakfast:** Anti-Inflammatory Breakfast Burritos
- **Lunch:** Balsamic Glazed Chicken and Roasted Vegetable Quinoa
- **Dinner:** Pineapple Teriyaki Chicken Skewers

Day 18:

- **Breakfast:** Kale, Pine Nut, and Raisin Breakfast Stir-Fry
- **Lunch:** Spicy Tofu Lettuce Wraps with Peanut Sauce
- **Dinner:** Artichoke and Spinach Stuffed Portobellos

Day 19:

- **Breakfast:** Mango and Turmeric Smoothie Bowl
- **Lunch:** Mediterranean Lentil and Spinach Soup
- **Dinner:** Vegan Paella with Saffron and Seasonal Vegetables

Day 20:

- **Breakfast:** Egg White, Spinach, and Mushroom Breakfast Wraps
- **Lunch:** Rainbow Vegetable and Hummus Tartine
- **Dinner:** Grilled Asparagus and Fennel Salad

Day 21:

- **Breakfast:** Savory Lentil and Sweet Potato Breakfast Bowl
- **Lunch:** Kale Caesar Salad with Grilled Chicken
- **Dinner:** Lemon Pepper Trout with Garlic Spinach

Week 4

Day 22:

- **Breakfast:** Whole Grain Toast with Avocado and Sprouts
- **Lunch:** Avocado, Tomato, and Cucumber Sushi Rolls
- **Dinner:** Roasted Brussels Sprouts with Pomegranate Glaze

Day 23:

- **Breakfast:** Spinach and Mushroom Egg Muffins
- **Lunch:** Tahini-Glazed Butternut Squash and Red Onion
- **Dinner:** Carrot Ginger Soup with Turmeric

Day 24:

- **Breakfast:** Avocado Berry Smoothie Bowl
- **Lunch:** Asian Quinoa Salad with Baked Teriyaki Salmon
- **Dinner:** Baked Cod with Lemon and Dill

Day 25:

- **Breakfast:** Sweet Potato Toast with Avocado Mash
- **Lunch:** Spinach and Mushroom Stuffed Sweet Potatoes
- **Dinner:** Eggplant Parmesan with Cashew Cheese

Day 26:

- **Breakfast:** Kale and Quinoa Breakfast Salad
- **Lunch:** Broccoli Quinoa Casserole with Chicken
- **Dinner:** Ratatouille with Quinoa Pilaf

Day 27:

- **Breakfast:** Smoked Salmon and Avocado Wrap
- **Lunch:** Mexican Quinoa Salad with Lime Cilantro Dressing
- **Dinner:** Spaghetti Squash with Tomato Basil Sauce

Day 28:

- **Breakfast:** Walnut and Pumpkin Seed Granola
- **Lunch:** Rainbow Vegetable Stir-Fry with Tamari Sauce
- **Dinner:** Roasted Garlic Cauliflower Mash

Day 29:

- **Breakfast:** Zucchini and Carrot Pancakes
- **Lunch:** Cauliflower Rice Tabbouleh with Grilled Chicken (repeat from Day 8 for variety)
- **Dinner:** Cilantro Lime Chicken with Avocado Salsa

Day 30:

- **Breakfast:** Buckwheat and Blueberry Porridge
- **Lunch:** Beetroot, Goat Cheese, and Arugula Salad with Roasted Beets (repeat from Day 12 for nutritional balance)
- **Dinner:** Moroccan Vegetable Tagine (repeat from Day 5 to end on a diverse note)

This comprehensive 30-day meal plan offers a diverse range of meals designed to reduce inflammation and introduce the foundational principles of an anti-inflammatory diet. Each week builds on the variety and complexity of meals, encouraging beginners to explore new flavors and ingredients. The key to a successful anti-inflammatory diet is variety, balance, and consistency. Enjoy discovering how these meals can contribute to improved health and well-being.

Shopping List

Creating a comprehensive shopping list for the 30-day meal plan involves consolidating ingredients from each recipe into categories such as fruits, vegetables, proteins, grains, etc. This list aims to cover the range of ingredients needed for the meals outlined in the plan, assuming a household of one to two people. Adjust quantities based on your specific needs, the number of servings required, and the assumption that some pantry staples (like olive oil, salt, and pepper) are already available.

Fruits:

- Avocados (15-20, depending on size)
- Mixed berries (fresh or frozen, 4 cups)
- Lemons (10-15)
- Limes (5-10)
- Mangoes (2-3)
- Apples (6-8)
- Pomegranates (2-3 or pre-seeded equivalent)
- Bananas (4-6)
- Pineapple (canned or fresh for 2 meals)
- Oranges for citrus vinaigrette (2-3)
- Cherries (fresh or frozen, for compote, if desired)
- Peaches (for baking, 2-3)

Vegetables:

- Sweet potatoes (6-8)
- Kale bunches (4-6)
- Spinach (4 large bags or bundles)
- Arugula (2 bags or bundles)
- Broccoli (4 heads or equivalent in florets)
- Mixed vegetables for roasting (zucchini, bell peppers, onions, etc., 8-10 cups total)
- Cauliflower (2 large heads)
- Butternut squash (2 medium)
- Eggplants (2-3)
- Zucchini (4-6)
- Carrots (1 bag, 1-2 lbs)
- Beets (3-4 large or pre-cooked equivalent)
- Mushrooms (2 kg)
- Garlic (1 bulb)
- Ginger (1 large piece)
- Cucumber (2-3)
- Cherry tomatoes (2 pints)
- Fennel (1-2 bulbs)

Proteins:

- Chicken breasts or thighs (6-8 pounds, considering multiple meals)

- Salmon fillets (4-6, depending on size)
- Eggs (2-3 dozen)
- Tofu (2-3 blocks)
- Lentils (red and green, 2 lbs each)
- Chickpeas (canned or dry, 2 kg)
- Black beans (canned or dry, 2 kg)
- Quinoa (2 kg)
- Shrimp (1-2 kg)
- Cod or any white fish (1-2 kg)
- Turkey (smoked or fresh, 1-2 kg)

Grains & Nuts:

- Buckwheat (1 lb)
- Whole grain noodles or pasta (1-2 packages)
- Farro (1 lb)
- Whole grain or sprouted grain bread (1 loaf)
- Walnuts, almonds, pumpkin seeds (1 lb each)
- Brown rice (1 lb)

Dairy & Alternatives:

- Coconut yogurt (for multiple servings)
- Feta cheese (1 block or pre-crumbled)
- Cashew cheese or any vegan cheese (if making vegan options)

Miscellaneous:

- Olive oil, coconut oil
- Vinegar (balsamic, apple cider)
- Tahini (1 jar)
- Spices: Turmeric, Cumin, Chili powder, Paprika, Cinnamon, Nutmeg, Ground ginger, Dill, Mint, Sea salt, Black pepper
- Honey, Maple syrup
- Chia seeds, Hemp seeds, Flaxseeds
- Soba noodles (1 package)
- Sushi nori wraps (for sushi rolls)
- Coconut milk (canned, 2-3)
- Tamari sauce or gluten-free soy sauce

Fresh Herbs:

- Cilantro
- Parsley
- Rosemary
- Thyme

Conclusion

As we close the pages of this cookbook, it's essential to reflect on the journey we've embarked upon together. Beginning with the fundamentals of inflammation and the pivotal role diet plays in managing it, we've traversed through the principles and practices of an anti-inflammatory lifestyle. From understanding the basics to stocking your kitchen, from savoring every meal to integrating essential lifestyle changes, this guide has aimed to be your compass in navigating the vast and sometimes complex world of anti-inflammatory eating.

The recipes, meal plans, and shopping lists provided were designed to introduce you to many flavors and nutrients and simplify what may initially seem like an overwhelming shift in dietary habits. By focusing on whole grains, fruits, vegetables, and anti-inflammatory proteins, we've laid a foundation that supports your health, combats inflammation and brings joy to your dining experience.

Incorporating physical activity, managing stress, and ensuring quality sleep support the dietary aspect of an anti-inflammatory lifestyle. These components work synergistically, enhancing the diet's benefits and contributing to a holistic approach to reducing inflammation and improving overall well-being.

As you continue this path, remember that the health journey is not linear. There will be challenges and successes, and tracking your progress, celebrating your achievements, and learning from every step is essential. This cookbook was designed to be a starting point, providing the tools and knowledge to make informed choices and adapt the anti-inflammatory diet to fit your unique needs and preferences.

Embrace this journey with an open heart and mind. Let the principles of anti-inflammatory eating guide you, but also allow yourself the flexibility to explore and enjoy the diversity of foods and flavors that contribute to your health. Here's to a future where every meal is nourishing for the body and a step toward vibrant health and vitality.

Thank you for allowing us to be a part of your journey to an anti-inflammatory lifestyle. May the path ahead be filled with discovery, health, and joy.

Made in the USA
Monee, IL
28 April 2024

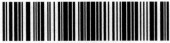

57625235R00085